Evidence-based Clinical Chinese Medicine

Volume 13
Post-Stroke Spasticity

Evidence-based Clinical Chinese Medicine

Co-Editors-in-Chief

Charlie Changli Xue
RMIT University, Australia

Chuanjian Lu
Guangdong Provincial Hospital of Chinese Medicine, China

Volume 13

Post-Stroke Spasticity

Lead Authors

Claire Shuiqing Zhang
RMIT University, Australia

Shaonan Liu
Guangdong Provincial Hospital of Chinese Medicine, China

World Scientific

NEW JERSEY • LONDON • SINGAPORE • BEIJING • SHANGHAI • HONG KONG • TAIPEI • CHENNAI • TOKYO

Published by

World Scientific Publishing Co. Pte. Ltd.
5 Toh Tuck Link, Singapore 596224
USA office: 27 Warren Street, Suite 401-402, Hackensack, NJ 07601
UK office: 57 Shelton Street, Covent Garden, London WC2H 9HE

Library of Congress Cataloging-in-Publication Data
Names: Xue, Charlie Changli, author. | Lu, Chuan-jian, 1964– author.
Title: Evidence-based clinical Chinese medicine / Charlie Changli Xue, Chuanjian Lu.
Description: New Jersey : World Scientific, 2016. | Includes bibliographical references and index.
Identifiers: LCCN 2015030389| ISBN 9789814723084 (v. 1 : hardcover : alk. paper) |
ISBN 9789814723091 (v. 1 : paperback : alk. paper) |
ISBN 9789814723121 (v. 2 : hardcover : alk. paper) |
ISBN 9789814723138 (v. 2 : paperback : alk. paper) |
ISBN 9789814759045 (v. 3 : hardcover : alk. paper) |
ISBN 9789814759052 (v. 3 : paperback : alk. paper)
Subjects: | MESH: Medicine, Chinese Traditional--methods. | Clinical Medicine--methods. |
Evidence-Based Medicine--methods. | Psoriasis. | Pulmonary Disease, Chronic Obstructive.
Classification: LCC RC81 | NLM WB 55.C4 | DDC 616--dc23
LC record available at http://lccn.loc.gov/2015030389

Volume 13: Post-Stroke Spasticity
ISBN 978-981-121-371-7 (hardcover)
ISBN 978-981-121-372-4 (ebook for institutions)
ISBN 978-981-121-373-1 (ebook for individuals)

British Library Cataloguing-in-Publication Data
A catalogue record for this book is available from the British Library.

For any available supplementary material, please visit
https://www.worldscientific.com/worldscibooks/10.1142/11650#t=suppl

Disclaimer

The information in this book is based on systematic analyses of the best available evidence for Chinese medicine interventions both historical and contemporary. Every effort has been made to ensure accuracy and completeness of the data of this publication. This book is intended for clinicians, researchers and educators. The practice of evidence-based medicine consists of consideration of the best available evidence, practitioners' clinical experience and judgment, and patients' preference. Not all interventions are acceptable in all countries. It is important to note that some of the substances mentioned in this book may no longer be in use, may be toxic, or may be prohibited or restricted under the provisions of the Convention on International Trade in Endangered Species of Wild Fauna and Flora (CITES). Practitioners, researchers and educators are advised to comply with the relevant regulations in their country and with the restrictions on the trade in species included in CITES appendices I, II and III. This book is not intended as a guide for self-medication. Patients should seek professional advice from qualified Chinese medicine practitioners.

Foreword

Since the late 20th century, Chinese medicine, including acupuncture and herbal medicine, has been increasingly used throughout the world. The parallel development and spread of evidence-based medicine has provided challenges and opportunities for Chinese medicine. The opportunities have been evidence-based medicine's emphasis on the effective use of the best available clinical evidence, incorporating the clinicians' clinical experience, subject to patients' preference. Such practices have a patient focus which reflects the historical nature of Chinese medicine practice. However, the challenges are also significant due to the fact that, despite the long-term development and very rich literature accumulated over 2,000 years, there is an overall lack of high-level clinical evidence for many of the interventions used in Chinese medicine.

To address this knowledge gap, we need to generate clinical evidence through high-quality clinical studies and to evaluate evidence to enable effective use of such available evidence to promote evidence-based Chinese medicine practice.

Modern Chinese medicine is rooted in its classical literature and the legacies of ancient doctors, grounded in the practice of expert clinicians and increasingly informed by clinical and experimental research efforts. In recognition of the unique features of Chinese medicine, for each of the conditions in this series a 'whole-evidence' approach is used to provide a synthesis of different types and levels of evidence to enable practitioners to make clinical decisions informed by the current best evidence.

There are four main components of this 'whole-evidence' approach. In the first component, we present the current approaches to the diagnosis, differentiation and treatment of each condition based on expert consensus of textbooks and clinical guidelines. This provides an overview of how the condition is currently managed. The second component provides an analysis of the condition in historical context based on systematic searches of the *Zhong Hua Yi Dian* which includes the full texts of more than 1,000 classical medical books. These analyses provide objective views on how the condition has been treated over two millennia, reveal continuities and discontinuities between traditional and modern practice, and suggest avenues for future research.

The third component is the assessment of evidence derived from modern clinical studies of Chinese medicine interventions. The methods established by the *Cochrane Collaboration* are used as the basis for conducting systematic reviews and undertaking meta-analyses of outcome data for randomised controlled trials (RCTs). In addition, the clinical relevance of meta-analysis data is enhanced by examining the herbal formulas, individual herbs and acupuncture treatments that were assessed in the RCTs, and the evidence base is broadened by the inclusion of data from controlled clinical trials and non-controlled studies. The fourth component is to determine how the herbal medicine interventions may achieve the effects indicated by the clinical trials. Thus for each of the most frequently used herbs we provide reviews of their effects in pre-clinical models and their likely mechanisms of action.

For each condition, this 'whole-evidence' approach links clinical expertise, historical precedent, clinical research data and experimental research to provide the reader with assessments of the current state of the evidence for the efficacy, effevtiveness and safety for Chinese medicine interventions using herbal medicines, acupuncture and moxibustion, and other health care practices such as *tuina*.

Since these books are available in Chinese and English, they can benefit patients, practitioners and educators internationally and enable practitioners to make clinical decisions informed by the current best evidence.

These publications represent a major milestone in the development of Chinese medicine and make a significant contribution to the development of evidence-based Chinese medicine globally.

Co-editors-in-Chief

Distinguished Professor Charlie Changli Xue
RMIT University, Australia

Professor Chuanjian Lu
Guangdong Provincial Hospital of Chinese Medicine, China

Purpose of This Book

This book is intended for clinicians, researchers and educators. It can be used to inform tertiary education and clinical practice by providing systematic, multi-dimensional assessments of the best available evidence for using Chinese medicine to manage each common clinical condition.

How to Use This Book

Some Definitions

A glossary is included, containing terms and definitions which frequently appear in the book. It also describes the definitions of statistical tests, methodological terms, evaluation tools and interventions. For example, in this book, integrative medicine refers to the combined use of a Chinese medicine treatment with conventional medical management, and combination therapies refer to two or more Chinese medicines from different therapy groups (e.g. Chinese herbal medicine, acupuncture or other Chinese medicine therapies) administered together. Terminology used throughout the book is based on the World Health Organisation's *Standard Terminologies on Traditional Medicine in the Western Pacific Region* (2007) where possible or from the cited reference.

Data Analysis and Interpretation of Results

In order to synthesise the clinical evidence, a range of statistical analysis approaches are used. In general, the effect size for dichotomous data is reported as a risk ratio (RR) with 95% confidence intervals (CI), and for continuous data, they are reported as mean difference (MD) with 95% (CI). Statistically significant effects are indicated with an asterisk*. Readers should note that statistically significant does not necessarily correspond with a clinically important effect. Interpretation of results should take into consideration of the clinical significance, quality of studies (expressed as high, low or unclear risk of bias in this book) and heterogeneity amongst the studies. Tests for heterogeneity are conducted using the I^2 statistic. An I^2 score greater than 50% was considered to indicate substantial heterogeneity.

Use of Evidence in Practice

The Grading of Recommendations Assessment, Development and Evaluation (GRADE) approach was used to summarise the certainty of the evidence for critical and important comparisons and outcomes. Due to the diverse nature of Chinese medicine practice, treatment recommendations are not included with the summary of findings tables. Therefore readers will need to interpret the evidence with reference to the local practice environment.

Limitations

Readers should note some of the methodological limitations on classical literature and clinical evidence.

- Search terms used to search the *Zhong Hua Yi Dian* database may not include all terms that have been used for the condition, which may alter the findings.
- Chinese language has changed over time. Citations have been interpreted for analysis, and such interpretations may be subject to disagreement.
- Chinese medicine theory has evolved over time. As such, concepts described in classical Chinese medical literature may no longer be found in contemporary works.

- Symptoms described in citations may be common to many conditions, and a judgment was required to determine the likelihood of the citation being related to the condition. This may have introduced some bias due to the subjective nature of the judgment.
- The vast majority of the clinical evidence for Chinese medicine treatments has come from China. The applicability of the findings to other populations and other countries requires further assessment.
- Many studies included participants with varying disease severity. Where possible, subgroup analyses were undertaken to examine the effects in different subpopulations. As this was not always possible, the findings may be limited to the population included, and not to subpopulations.
- The potential risk of bias found in many included studies suggested methodological limitations. The findings for GRADE assessments based on studies of very low- to moderate-certainty evidence should be interpreted accordingly.
- Nine major English- and Chinese-language databases were searched to identify clinical studies, in addition to clinical trial registers. Other studies may exist which were not identified through searches, and which may alter the findings.
- The calculation of frequency of herbal formula use was based on formula names only. It is possible that studies evaluated herbal treatments with the same or similar herb ingredients, but which were given different formula names. Due to the complexity of herbal formulas, it was considered not appropriate to make a judgment as to the similarity of formulas for analysis. As such, the frequency of formulas reported in Chapter 5 may be underestimated.
- The most frequent utilised herbs which may have contributed to the treatment effect have been described in Chapter 5. These herbs may provide leads for further exploration. Calculation of the herbs with potential effect is based on frequency of formulas reported in the studies, and does not take into consideration the clinical implications and functions of every herb in a formula.

Authors and Contributors

Co-editors-in-Chief

Prof. Charlie Changli Xue (*RMIT University, Australia*)
Prof. Chuanjian Lu (*Guangdong Provincial Hospital of Chinese Medicine, China*)

Co-deputy Editors-in-Chief

Assoc. Prof. Anthony Lin Zhang (*RMIT University, Australia*)
Dr. Brian H May (*RMIT University, Australia*)
Prof. Xinfeng Guo (*Guangdong Provincial Hospital of Chinese Medicine, China*)
Prof. Zehuai Wen (*Guangdong Provincial Hospital of Chinese Medicine, China*)

Lead Authors

Dr. Claire Shuiqing Zhang (*RMIT University, Australia*)
Dr. Shaonan Liu (*Guangdong Provincial Hospital of Chinese Medicine, China*)

Co-Authors

RMIT University (Australia):
Dr. Xinmei Zhang
Assoc. Prof. Anthony Lin Zhang
Prof. Charlie Changli Xue

Guangdong Provincial Hospital of Chinese Medicine (China):
Dr. Yiyi Cai
Dr. Ruihuan Pan

Prof. Youhua Guo
Prof. Hongxia Chen
Prof. Xinfeng Guo
Prof. Zehuai Wen
Prof. Chuanjian Lu

Members of Advisory Committee and Panel

Co-chairs of Project Planning Committee

Prof. Peter J Coloe (*RMIT University, Australia*)
Prof. Yubo Lyu (*Guangdong Provincial Hospital of Chinese Medicine, China*)
Prof. Dacan Chen (*Guangdong Provincial Hospital of Chinese Medicine, China*)

Centre Advisory Committee (in Alphabetical Order)

Prof. Keji Chen (*The Chinese Academy of Sciences, China*)
Prof. Aiping Lu (*Hong Kong Baptist University, China*)
Prof. Caroline Smith (*University of Western Sydney, Australia*)
Prof. David F Story (*RMIT University, Australia*)

Methodology Expert Advisory Panel (in Alphabetical Order)

Prof. Zhaoxiang Bian (*Hong Kong Baptist University, China*)
The late Prof. George Lewith (*University of Southampton, United Kingdom*)
Prof. Lixing Lao (The University of Hong Kong, China)
Prof. Jianping Liu (*Beijing University of Chinese Medicine, China*)
Prof. Frank Thien (*Monash University, Australia*)
Prof. Jialiang Wang (*Sichuan University, China*)

Content Expert Advisory Panel (in Alphabetical Order)

Prof. Jongbae Jay Park (*Department of Anesthesiology Center for Translational Pain Medicine, Duke University, US*)

Prof. Linpeng Wang (*Beijing Hospital of Chinese Medicine, China*)
Prof. Zehuai Wen (*Guangdong Provincial Hospital of Chinese Medicine, China*)
Prof. Fang Zeng (*Chengdu University of Chinese Medicine, China*)
Prof. Guoqing Zheng (*The Second Affiliation Hospital of Wenzhou Medical University, China*)

Distinguished Professor Charlie Changli Xue

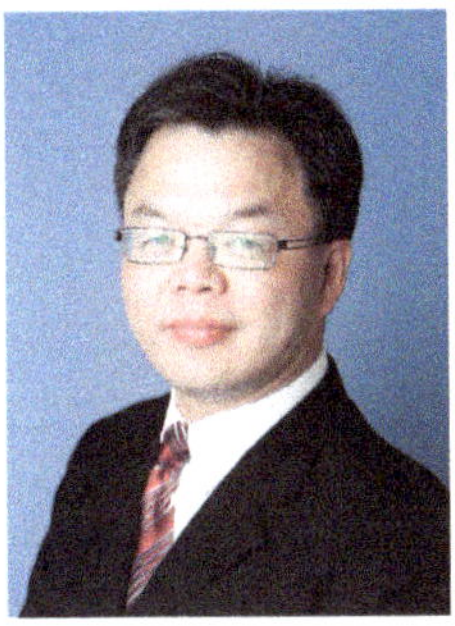

Distinguished Professor Charlie Changli Xue holds a Bachelor of Medicine (majoring in Chinese Medicine) from Guangzhou University of Chinese Medicine, China (1987) and a PhD from RMIT University, Australia (2000). He has been an academic, researcher, regulator and practitioner for almost three decades. Professor Xue has made significant contributions to evidence-based educational development, clinical research, regulatory framework and policy development, and provision of high-quality clinical care to the community. Professor Xue is recognised internationally as an expert in evidence-based traditional medicine and integrative health care.

Professor Xue is the Inaugural National Chair of the Chinese Medicine Board of Australia appointed by the Australian Health Workforce Ministerial Council (in 2011), and he was reappointed for a second term in 2014. Since 2007, he has been a Member of the World Health Organisation (WHO) Expert Advisory Panel for Traditional and Complementary Medicine, Geneva. Professor Xue is also Honorary Senior Principal Research Fellow at the Guangdong Provincial Academy of Chinese Medical Sciences, China.

At RMIT, Professor Xue is Executive Dean, School of Health and Biomedical Sciences. He is also Director of the WHO Collaborating Centre for Traditional Medicine.

Between 1995 and 2010, Professor Xue was Discipline Head of Chinese Medicine at RMIT University. He leads the development of five successful undergraduate and postgraduate degree programmes in Chinese Medicine at RMIT University which is now a global leader in Chinese medicine education and research.

Professor Xue's research has been supported by research grants of over AUD 15 million, including six project grants from the Australian Government's National Health and Medical Research Council (NHMRC) and two Australian Research Council (ARC) grants. He has contributed over 200 publications and has been frequently invited as keynote speaker for numerous national and international conferences. Professor Xue has contributed to over 300 media interviews on issues related to complementary medicine education, research, regulation and practice.

Professor Chuanjian Lu

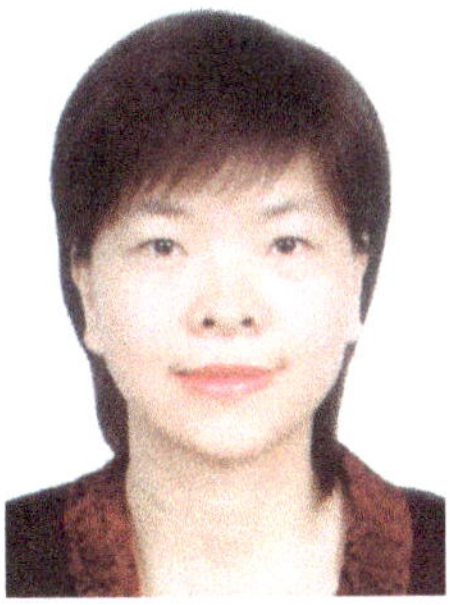

Professor Chuanjian Lu, Doctor of Medicine. She is the Vice-president of Guangdong Provincial Hospital of Chinese Medicine (Guangdong Provincial Academy of Chinese Medical Sciences, Second Clinical Medical College of Guangzhou University of Chinese Medicine). She also is the Chair of the Guangdong Traditional Chinese Medicine (TCM) Standardization Technical Committee, and the Vice-chair of the Immunity Specialty Committee of the World Federation of Chinese Medicine Societies (WFCMS).

Professor Lu has engaged in scientific research into TCM, clinical practice and teaching for some 25 years. Her research has been devoted to integrating traditional and western medicine. She has edited and published 12 monographs and 120 academic research articles as first author and corresponding author with over 30 articles being included in SCI journals.

She has received widespread recognition for her achievements with awards for Excellent Teacher of South China, National Outstanding Women TCM Doctor and National Outstanding Young Doctor of TCM. She also received the Science and Technology Star of the Association of Chinese Medicine, the National Excellent Science and Technology Workers of China Award and the Five-continent Women's Scientific Awards of China Medical Women's Association.

Professor Lu has won the Award of Science and Technology Progress over ten times from Guangdong Provincial Government, China Association of Chinese Medicine and Chinese Hospital Association.

Acknowledgements

The authors and contributors would like to acknowledge the valuable contributions of research assistants and students who assisted with database searches, data extraction, data screening, data assessment, translation of documents, editing and/or administrative tasks: Ms. Yiran Ai, Dr. Jhodie Duncan, Ms. Aiping Li, Ms. Ruzhuang Liang, Ms. Jingmin Lu, Dr. George Shengxi Zhang, Ms. Jingwen Zhu, Ms. Ke Zhu and Mr. Jinhong Zuo.

Contents

List of Figures

List of Tables

1

Introduction to Post-stroke Spasticity

OVERVIEW

Spasticity is one of the most commonly seen motor-function complications after stroke; it can adversely impact on stroke survivors and worsen other post-stroke complications. Spasticity could be a great barrier in the rehabilitation process of stroke recovery. This chapter reviews the definition, epidemiology, classification, diagnosis, prognosis and clinical management of post-stroke spasticity.

Introduction

Stroke was defined as 'developing clinical signs of focal (or global) disturbance of cerebral function, with symptoms lasting 24 hours, or longer, or leading to death, with no apparent cause other than of vascular origin' by the World Health Organisation (WHO) in 1989.[1] Ischaemic stroke caused by the arterial and venous systems, intracerebral haemorrhage, and subarachnoid haemorrhage are the three common vascular origins.

According to the reports of the WHO on stroke epidemiology, around 6.7 million deaths were attributed to stroke in 2012. Hence, it is considered the third most common cause of death in developed countries, exceeded only by coronary heart disease and cancer.[2] Despite the high mortality rate, it has been estimated that around 40% of stroke patients were left with moderate functional impairments and 15–30% with severe disability.[3,4] Worldwide, 15 million people suffer a stroke each year; one-third die and one-third are left permanently disabled.[2] The rates of stroke mortality and burden vary greatly among countries.[5] In Australia, stroke is one of the biggest killers and a leading cause of disability. It was reported that, in 2012, there were over 420,000 people living with the effects of stroke,[6] and the total financial costs of stroke in Australia in 2012 were estimated to be AUD 5 billion.[7] The prevalence of stroke in China is higher than in other developing countries, and it has been increasing in recent years. In China, with the current 1.4 billion population, the annual stroke mortality rate is approximately 1.6 million (around 157 per 100,000), which has exceeded heart disease to become the leading cause of death and adult disability. In addition, China has 2.5 million new stroke cases each year and 7.5 million stroke survivors.[8,9] Stroke causes a significant financial burden in China. It was reported that the annual direct cost of stroke care in China is approximately ten times higher than the care cost associated with cardiovascular diseases.[10,11]

Effective rehabilitation interventions initiated early after stroke can enhance the recovery process and the quality of life, and minimise functional disability. Improved functional outcomes for patients also contribute to patient satisfaction and reduce potential costly long-term care expenditures. The primary goals of rehabilitation are to prevent complications, minimise impairments and maximise function.[12]

Certain post-stroke complications have a substantial effect on the final outcome of patients with stroke and often impede neurological recovery. Post-stroke complications can be summarised as the following categories:

- Motor function complications: Include muscle spasticity (an abnormal increase in muscle tone), joint contractures and shoulder problems;
- Cognitive and psychological complications: Range from mild impairment of mental processes to severe dementia causing disability;
- Complications due to immobility: Following a stroke, patients may have limited mobility which predisposes them to complications such as pressure sores and deep vein thrombosis;

- Nutrition: Stroke patients often have swallowing difficulties which can increase the risk of choking and chest infection, hence reducing nutrition intake;
- Infections: Stroke patients are at risk of infections, particularly those affecting the chest and urinary tract;
- Disuse syndrome or misuse syndrome.

Among these, spasticity is one of the most commonly seen motor function problems after stroke. It contributes to the impairments and disabilities that negatively impact functional recovery. This chapter summarises the definition, epidemiology, diagnosis, assessment of severity and treatments of post-stroke spasticity, according to current clinical guidelines.

Definition of Post-stroke Spasticity

Spasticity was traditionally defined in 1980 as 'a motor disorder characterised by a velocity-dependent increase in tonic stretch reflexes (muscle tone) with exaggerated tendon jerks resulting from hyper-excitability of the stretch reflex as one component of the upper motor neuron syndrome',[13] with an emphasis on the difficulty of passive movement and no consideration of the voluntary gestures. In 1994, neurophysiological factors were added to the definition of spasticity as 'a motor disorder characterised by a velocity-dependent increase in tonic stretch reflexes that results from abnormal intra-spinal processing of primary afferent input'.[14] In 2005, the definition of spasticity was further modified as 'a disordered sensorimotor control, resulting from an upper motor neuron lesion, presenting as intermittent or sustained involuntary activation of muscles'.[15] Currently there is no universal and consistent definition of post-stroke spasticity, which probably indicates the complexity and diversity of its manifestations and underlying mechanisms. Spasticity is one of the most significant impairments for stroke survivors, which may lead to body pain, problems with skin hygiene, and most severely, contractures that render the affected limb functionless and spastic equinovarus foot.[12]

Clinical Presentation of Post-stroke Spasticity

Post-stroke patients usually develop a group of symptoms and signs that constitute the upper motor neuron syndrome.[16] Spasticity is characterised by increased muscle tone, exaggerated tendon jerks and poor control of voluntary movement that occurs as a component of an upper motor neuron syndrome. Other components include tendon hyper-reflexia, clonus, the clasp-knife phenomenon, flexor and extensor spasms, a Babinski sign and spastic dystonia.

Although the exact natural history of how spasticity develops currently is unknown, there are symptoms and signs that are observed as clinical characteristics in stroke survivors indicating spasticity. The typical feature of spasticity is the high muscle tone that varies with the speed of movement, where the resistance becomes greater if the stretch goes faster. It is said that the resistance is 'felt like a catch after an initial few degrees of movement'.[17] In most cases, the manifestations of post-stroke spasticity are not presented alone, but more commonly, it is accompanied by other dysfunctions or changes of motor function.

Clinical Characteristics of the Upper Limbs with Spasticity

In the upper limbs of stroke survivors with spasticity, the antigravity muscle groups are characteristically affected by the increased muscle tone, which is usually high in the adductors of the shoulders, flexors of elbows, wrists and fingers, as well as the pronators of the forearm. Furthermore, the typical clenched fist with 'thumb in palm' deformity is supposed to be the result from excessive flexion of fingers and adduction of the thumb.[17]

Spasticity is also the inevitable accompaniment of hemiplegia and an incomplete motor recovery,[16] among which hemiplegic shoulder pain is directly linked with abnormal muscle tone. Two commonly seen conditions for hemiplegic shoulder pain related to spasticity are *subscapularis spasticity disorder* and *pectoralis spasticity disorder*. The subscapularis spasticity disorder is characterised by motion being most limited and pain being reproduced on external rotation.[18] As for the pectoralis spasticity disorder, it is characterised by motion being most limited and pain produced on abduction.

Clinical Characteristics of the Lower Limbs with Spasticity

In terms of the lower limbs, spasticity causes the high tone in adductors of the hip, flexors of the knee and plantar, and invertors of the ankle. Due to persistent high tone of extensor hallucis longus, the hyperextension of the big toe is another characteristic of spasticity, which may cause difficulty in using footwear for patients.[17]

The adductor with spasticity, resulting in the plantar flexion and inversion at the knee, forms part of the lower limb pattern in hemiplegia, pulls the knees together and at the ankles limits the range of movement. In addition, spasticity of the gastrocnemius and tibialis posterior muscles is a common cause of spastic equinovarus foot after stroke, making patients suffer deformity and difficulty with gait. Moreover, observation of the paretic limbs shows that the paretic limbs with muscle spasticity are at considerably high risk of developing contractures, which not only limit the movement of the involved joints, but also lead to significant pain.[18]

Complications or Coexisting Disorders

It is believed that post-stroke spasticity can also induce changes in rheological muscle properties, such as stiffness, fibrosis and atrophy.[19] Meanwhile, spasticity is associated with several complications, including falls, pain, pressure ulcers, infections and contractures.[17]

Epidemiology of Post-stroke Spasticity

Since the incidence of post-stroke spasticity is not always reported separately, its prevalence may be underestimated even though spasticity is considered one of the most commonly seen complications after stroke [20,21] affecting around 20–50% of survivors.[22–25] However, there is a variation in the onset time of spasticity after stroke, which in turn may have an impact on measuring the prevalence of post-stroke spasticity. Related evidence shows that at the early stage (zero to three months) after stroke, the occurrence rate of spasticity is between 19% and 28%.[24] The percentage of survivors suffering spasticity increases slightly to 43% during the medium term (three months to one year) after stroke.[26] Regarding the long-term phase after stroke (longer than one year), the prevalence of spasticity is between 17% and 46%.[23,27,28]

Burden of Post-stroke Spasticity

Firstly, spastic symptoms can induce pain, ankylosis, tendon retraction or muscle weakness in patients, which may limit the potential success of rehabilitation.[12,29] Moreover, poor posture may result in difficulty in changes and transfers in position. Therefore, patients with severe spasticity may suffer from hygiene problems, including cleaning of the hands, axillae, elbows and especially genital areas. Besides bowel and bladder care, spasticity may also interfere with sexual relationships.[17] Hence, stroke survivors with spasticity suffer not only the negative physical effects, but also the psychological and social impacts on life.[30]

In terms of the financial burden, it has been reported that the direct cost for patients with post-stroke spasticity is nearly four times that of stroke survivors without spasticity.[26] The long-term financial burden of post-stroke spasticity increases the costs for both the family and society. It should be noted that, due to the consequences and co-morbidities following post-stroke spasticity (such as falls, fractures, etc.), it not only requires a higher treatment cost, but also increases caregiver burden.[31,32] Interestingly, it is not uncommon that spasticity sometimes serves as compensation for muscle weakness. For example, the stiffness of the weak muscles of the lower limbs can assist sitting, standing, transfers and walking, while spasticity of long finger flexor muscles helps patients to use implements like cutlery or a toothbrush.[17]

Risk Factors of Post-stroke Spasticity

Some factors are observed as possible risk factors for the development or progression of spasticity in stroke survivors. More evidence is needed to help confirm the relationship between these factors and post-stroke spasticity.[33] These include stroke lesions in the brainstem, haemorrhagic stroke, younger age, low Barthel Index at baseline, early arm or leg weakness, or paresis from days to 16 weeks, evidence of left-sided weakness, smoking, hemispasticity that occurs more often in the arm, more than two joints affected and a modified Ashworth Score of ≥ 2 from baseline to first follow-up (median time = six weeks).[28,34–37] Although these factors are suggested to predict disabling spasticity in post-stroke patients, they can hardly forecast the onset, severity and regional distribution of spasticity, nor can they indicate the different responses to therapies or rehabilitation measures.[33]

Furthermore, if patients with post-stroke spasticity worsen with aggravation of pain, stiffness, involuntary movements, deterioration of mobility, increase in care needs and sexual dysfunction, it is possible this results from the following three reasons: (1) triggers, (2) primary neurological disease progression, and (3) the occurrence and development of new diseases.[17] To identify the reasons of exacerbation of spasticity, one needs to look for any possible triggers first. If no underlying triggers are identified, then primary neurological disease progression and the occurrence and development of new diseases need to be considered.

Triggers for Worsening of Spasticity

Spasticity may be aggravated by triggers such as visceral or somatic stimuli below the level of injury.[37] The triggers for worsening of spasticity are listed below:

- Skin: Ulcers, ingrown toenails, boils and skin infections;
- Visceral: Constipation, urinary tract infections, urinary tract calculi and pain during menstruation;

- Devices: Improper seating, ill-fitting orthotics and failure of intrathecal baclofen pump;
- Drugs: Rapid withdrawal of anti-spasticity drugs;
- Others: Infections, injuries, deep vein thrombosis and stress.

Pathological Processes of Post-stroke Spasticity

Although the pathophysiologic basis of spasticity has not been completely understood, the following explanations were put forward to help understand the underlying mechanisms of the development of spasticity after stroke. Spasticity is one of the positive features of upper motor neuron syndrome, resulting from afferent-dependent abnormal spinal reflexes.[38] The occurrence of upper motor neuron syndrome is largely due to parapyramidal fibre dysfunction, with both excitatory and inhibitory pathways. The dorsal reticulospinal tract is the main tract inhibiting spinal reflex activity, while the excitatory neurons arise in the bulbopontine tegmentum, descending in the medial reticulospinal tract.[38]

Spinal reflexes seem to be the reason for the positive features of upper motor neuron syndrome, but how exactly they work in the development of spasticity remains unknown. Many changes could help explain the pathophysiology, such as decreased presynaptic inhibition, the failure of reciprocal inhibition from antagonistic muscles, decreased homosynaptic depression and changes of motor neuron properties.[33,38] During the process of spinal reflexes, it is the abnormal processing of proprioceptive input in the spinal cord, mediated by Ia afferents that seems to be the key to the development of spasticity, enhancing the central excitability.[38]

To some extent, the negative features of upper motor neuron syndrome, such as muscle weakness, may lead to muscle immobilisation at a short length and therefore, to hypertonia, stiffness and contracture, which in turn contribute to the development and worsening of spasticity.[38] However, the clinical presentation of post-stroke spasticity differs in terms of onset, severity and regional distribution, which suggests that there may be more than one mechanism underlying post-stroke spasticity.

Diagnosis of Post-stroke Spasticity

The symptoms of spasticity often seem obvious. An accurate diagnosis by an expert in neuromuscular disorders is essential for designing a treatment plan. When symptoms are mild, expert evaluation is even more important so that treatment is not delayed due to misdiagnosis. A complete physical examination, including neurological testing, will assess the extent of the spasticity. In addition to the medical and neurological exam, anyone with symptoms of spasticity should be evaluated by a physical therapist to determine which exact muscles are involved.[17]

Imaging tests may help provide information about the nature and extent of the brain damage causing the spasticity. For example, magnetic resonance imaging (MRI) scans produce detailed images of the brain and spine and allow doctors to see abnormalities that may cause spasticity.

Differential Diagnosis of Spasticity

As one of the most commonly seen complications in patients after stroke, spasticity usually occurs in combination with, and even in relation to, the development of other dysfunctions in stroke survivors. Therefore, the cut-off line to differentiate spasticity from other similar conditions following stroke may not be specified and clear enough, and so far no consensus has been reached with regard to the differential diagnosis of post-stroke spasticity.[17] Nair *et al.* (2014)[17] discussed three related, yet different conditions, whose typical feature is increased muscle tone. They are contractures, rigidity and catatonia.

Characterised by an abnormal shortening and reduction in the elasticity of tendons, muscles, joint capsules, ligaments and skin, contracture is accompanied by an increase in the resistance to passive stretch.[39,40] The difference between spasticity and contracture also lies in the dynamic changes of muscle tone with the speed of movement. But in post-stroke patients, contraction could also be one of the results of deterioration due to spasticity.

Table 1.1 Differential Diagnosis of Spasticity

	Spasticity	Contractures	Rigidity	Catatonia
Shortening tendons and muscles	No	Yes	No	No
Dynamic changes of muscle tone with speed of movement	Yes	No	No	No
Affects muscles selectively	Yes	No	No	No
Psychiatric factor involved	No	No	No	Yes
Waxy flexibility	No	No	No	Yes

Rigidity is related to pathological changes of the basal ganglia. Its increased muscle tone affects all muscles acting on a joint equally and therefore it is non-selective. But spasticity usually affects only certain muscle groups of a joint. In addition, rigidity can lead to resistance to passive movements throughout the whole range of movement without changing the speed.[17]

Catatonia is a neuropsychiatric syndrome that can be caused by several psychiatric, neurological and medical conditions, including stroke, phencyclidine intoxication and post-encephalitic Parkinsonism. It is featured by gegenhalten, abnormal posturing and 'waxy flexibility'. Unlike spasticity, patients with catatonia often present an increase in muscle tone proportional to the force applied.[41] The differences between spasticity and the abovementioned conditions are summarised in Table 1.1.

Moreover, clinical manifestations varied partly due to the combination of other signs of upper motor neuron syndrome. Table 1.2 summarises the six commonly seen features in upper motor neuron syndrome.[17]

Assessment of Patients with Spasticity

In general, the assessment of patients suffering spasticity includes focal muscle evaluation, as well as its impact on limb function and activity as a whole.

Table 1.2 Positive Signs of Upper Motor Neuron Syndrome

	Spasticity	Flexor Spasms	Clasp Knife Phenomenon	Spastic Dystonia	Associated Reactions	Co-contraction
Key features of clinical manifestation	Velocity-dependent increase in tonic stretch reflex.	A sudden stiffening of a muscle which may cause a limb to kick out or jerk towards your body.	A stretch reflex with a rapid decrease in resistance when attempting to flex a joint.	Continuous muscle contraction.	An involuntary movement of a body part associated with the resisted movement of another body part.	Simultaneous contraction of agonist and antagonist muscle groups.
Pathophysiology	Abnormal processing of proprioceptive input in the spinal cord.	Disinhibited afferents of normal flexor withdrawal reflexes.	Afferent-modified stretch reflex underlying spasticity.	Efferent-mediated tonic supraspinal drive to the α-motor neurons.	A failure to inhibit spread of motor activity through propriospinal pathways in the spinal cord.	Reduced or excessive reciprocal inhibition controlled at the cortical or spinal level.

Focal Muscle Evaluation

The basic assessment of spasticity mainly includes the neurological examination of muscle tone, motor power, reflexes and sensory level. Quantification through a validated scoring system is essential for the evaluation of spasticity. The most frequently used one is the Ashworth Scale (AS) or the Modified Ashworth Scale (MAS).[42,43]

Four other scales can also be used for the focal muscle evaluation for spasticity:

- Tardieu Scale and the Modified Tardieu Scale: Can be applied to the assessment of the passive range of motion, quality of muscle reaction to passive stretch at the fastest stretching velocity, and angle of muscle reaction at the point of resistance to the fastest stretching velocity when the overactive stretch reflex produces a first catch;[44–46]
- The Composite Spasticity Index (CSI): A measure for extremity spasticity. It is suitable for stroke survivors with hemiparesis by assessing the tendon jerk and clonus, and the tonic stretch reflex with assessment of resistance to passive movement of the limb;[47]
- Other less often used scales are developed by Priebe and Penn counting spasm frequency,[48,49] the Pendulum Test assessing the knee spasticity,[50,51] etc.

Assessment of Function and Activity

The scales mentioned above, however, are dependent on the examiner's impression of spasticity on passive movement and therefore, may be questioned sometimes on their reliability and validity.[52,53] Since post-stroke spasticity is often accompanied by other dysfunctions, or may lead to secondary complications, in order to get an overall understanding of the patient's situation, it is more meaningful to include multiple factors in the assessment including weakness, abnormal sensations and pain, as well as bladder, bowel, and sexual dysfunction and quality of life.

There are some scales that may give additional information, such as scales for activities of daily living (i.e. Barthel Index, Functional

Independence Measure), scores for limb function (Fugl-Meyer Assessment of Sensorimotor Recovery after Stroke, Motor Assessment Scale) and scales for neurologic outcome and degree of recovery for patients with stroke (i.e. National Institutes of Health Stroke Scale). These scales alone, however, are not sufficient for clinical assessment of spasticity.[54,55]

Management of Post-stroke Spasticity

Early initial rehabilitation is the key to preventing disabling complications. However, the exact intervention and initiation time for post-stroke spasticity prevention at an early stage following stroke remains unclear. Regarding the initial prevention and treatment of post-stroke spasticity, suggestions from clinical guidelines vary from mild spasticity to moderate or severe spasticity that interferes with the patients' mobility, activity of daily living and sleep, or that requires personal care.[12,16,18,20,56–61]

The general aim of therapy is to limit the impact of spasticity on stroke survivors and to prevent secondary complications. The goals of therapy include:[17]

- Relief of pain and discomfort;
- Improvement of posture;
- Facilitation of sitting, standing and walking;
- Reduction in burden of care;
- Improvement of hygiene in areas such as the palm, axilla and groin;
- Improvement in body image and self-esteem;
- Prevention of complications such as pressure ulcers.

In order to achieve these goals, a core multidisciplinary stroke rehabilitation team is needed and should comprise, but not be limited to, the following professional[57]:

- Consultant physicians;
- Nurses;
- Pharmacists;

- Physiotherapists;
- Speech and language therapists;
- Occupational therapists;
- Rehabilitation assistants;
- Social workers;
- Clinical psychologists;
- Dietitians;
- Orthoptists.

Therefore, due to the diversity and complexity of post-stroke dysfunctions and complications, rehabilitation programmes need to be individualised according to the patient's activity, care needs and access to physical therapy.[17] Moreover, long-term comprehensive therapies including pharmacologic and non-pharmacologic interventions are supposed to be beneficial for patients with spasticity.[57]

Recommendations from guidelines differ in therapeutic methods, their target users, as well as the intensity of rehabilitation. It is believed that interventions without physical therapy can only transiently reduce spasticity, but cannot result in functional gains.[18] Therefore, to combine pharmacological modalities that reduce spasticity with aggressive physical therapy is widely accepted. Besides indirect management, such as for infections, constipation and deep vein thrombosis, it is necessary to address or avoid the triggers that may exacerbate spasticity after stroke.[60]

Non-pharmacologic Therapies

Although physical therapies are the first-line treatment for post-stroke spasticity,[58] currently there is no reliable evidence indicating which physical therapy suits clinical needs the most with, or without, anti-spasticity medications.[18] Conventionally, a series of stepwise therapies are applied to the treatment of post-stroke spasticity with the most conservative forms at the beginning, such as positioning, then gradually progressing to less conservative ones, including passive stretching, range-of-motion exercises and corrective measures for contractures, including splinting, serial casting and surgical correction.[58] However, evidence for these therapies for post-stroke spasticity is inconclusive and even indicate conflicting effects.[62,63] In patients who already demonstrated contracture owing to spasticity, stretching using splints, machines or prolonged positioning may not be beneficial but sometimes more harmful with poor compliance and increased pain.[64–68]

As for electrical stimulation, studies also show different results.[69,70] Electromyogram (EMG) biofeedback seems effective in combination with electrical stimulation in reducing spasticity and is well tolerated during exercise.[71]

Pharmacologic Treatments

It is suggested that spasticity of the limbs in stroke survivors should not receive routine pharmacologic treatments, either orally or by injection, unless significant symptoms or interference with rehabilitation occurs.[58]

Oral Medications

Oral medications can be considered depending on the response of non-pharmacologic therapies. Evidence of oral medications for post-stroke spasticity treatment is limited and controversial, as the conclusions focus on spasticity and pain relief but functional benefits may be disappointing.[18,58] It is also suggested that such oral anti-spastic medication is associated with high levels of side effects.[72] The commonly used oral medications include baclofen, tizanidine and dantrolene. However, evidence for these medications is inclusive.[73,74]

As for diazepam and other benzodiazepines, due to their possible interference with cerebral functions that produces sedation that may reduce patients' ability to get involved in post-stroke rehabilitation effectively, they should be avoided during the stroke recovery period.[18]

Botulinum Toxin-A

Botulinum toxin-A may be used to target specific muscles or muscle groups;[60] it has proven effects on decreasing muscle tone and increasing active and passive range of motion in the limbs.[59] Strong evidence is also available suggesting that combing botulinum toxin-A injection and physiotherapy can improve extremity function.[75–78] Moreover, botulinum toxin-A seems well tolerated with no severe adverse events reported.[59]

However, the clinical effect of botulinum toxin-A is usually limited and lasts only two to three months, with a relatively high price.[58] Moreover, its impacts on activity level and change in quality of life are less well studied.[79,80] With regard to shoulder spasticity and pain, results from several randomised controlled trials (RCTs) even show conflicting conclusions.[81–85] The indication for use of botulinum toxin-A is mainly targeting patients with moderate to severe upper limb spasticity after stroke, whose MAS scores are no less than 3, as a second-line therapy when standard management has failed or as an adjunct to physiotherapy.[59]

Intrathecal Baclofen

For severe spastic hemiplegia, intrathecal baclofen could be an option.[86] It has been shown that intrathecal baclofen could be beneficial for chronic stroke patients with spasticity in small-sized clinical trials.[87] However, adverse events related to the therapy was also reported in a small proportion of cases.[88,89]

Neurosurgical Procedure

Another option for severe spasticity is neurosurgical procedure, although current evidence from clinical trials does not support routine application of neurosurgical therapies, such as selective dorsal rhizotomy or dorsal root entry zone lesions, in stroke survivors. It is rarely used in clinical practice probably because of the significant risks of these invasive treatments, including operative complications and unintended spinal cord damage.[12]

Chinese Medicine Therapies for Post-stroke Spasticity

Chinese medicine therapies including acupuncture, Chinese herbal medicine (CHM), acupuncture and therapeutic massage (*tuina* 推拿)

therapy have been commonly practised in China, and in recent years also in Western countries, for the management of post-stroke complications. Clinical researches investigating the efficacy and safety of these therapies have shown promising benefit when they were used for post-stroke spasticity.[90–95]

Prognosis of Post-stroke Spasticity

Left untreated, spasticity can have a devastating effect on physical function, activity and comfort. It can have a large impact on care delivery and participation restrictions in daily living, and may even lead to musculoskeletal complications, such as contracture.[20,38] The prognosis will vary significantly depending on spasticity location, access to post-stroke management and compliance to the rehabilitation plan.

A summary of this chapter can be seen in Table 1.3.

Table 1.3 Chapter Summary

Definition	• Disordered sensorimotor control, resulting from an upper motor neuron lesion, presenting as intermittent or sustained involuntary activation of muscles; • Spasticity is one of the most significant impairments for stroke survivors, which may lead to body pain, problems with skin hygiene and most severely, contractures that render the affected limb functionless and spastic equinovarus foot.
Main characteristics	• Spasticity is characterised by increased muscle tone, exaggerated tendon jerks and poor control of voluntary movement. Other components include tendon hyper-reflexia, clonus, the clasp-knife phenomenon, flexor and extensor spasms, a Babinski sign and spastic dystonia.
Diagnosis	• Based on symptoms and a complete physical examination including neurological testing.
Management	• Physical therapies; • Electrical stimulation; • Botulinum toxin-A; • Neurosurgical procedure.
Pharmacological management	• Baclofen, tizanidine and dantrolene.

References

1. World Health Organization. (1989) Recommendations on stroke prevention, diagnosis, and therapy. Report of the WHO Task Force on Stroke and other Cerebrovascular Disorders. *Stroke* **20(10):** 1407–1431.
2. World Health Organization. (2014) Global status report on noncommunicable diseases. Available from: http://www.who.int/nmh/publications/ncd-status-report-2014/en/.
3. American Heart Association. (2011) Heart and stroke statistical update 2011. American Heart Association, Dallas, TX.
4. Winstein CJ, Stein J, Arena R, *et al.* (2016) Guidelines for adult stroke rehabilitation and recovery: A guideline for healthcare professionals from the American Heart Association/American Stroke Association. American Heart Association Stroke Council, Council on Cardiovascular and Stroke Nursing, Council on Clinical Cardiology, and Council on Quality of Care and Outcomes Research. *Stroke* **47(6):** e98–e169.
5. Johnston SC, Mendis S, Mathers CD. (2009) Global variation in stroke burden and mortality: Estimates from monitoring, surveillance, and modelling. *Lancet Neurol* **8(4):** 345–354.
6. Australian Institute of Health and Welfare. (2012) Australia's health 2012. Australia's health series no.13. Cat. no. AUS 156. Canberra: AIHW. Available from: https://www.aihw.gov.au.
7. National Stroke Foundation. (2013) The economic impact of stroke in Australia. Available from: file://rmit.internal/USRHome/el6/E77936/Downloads/Final-Deloitte-Stroke-Report-14-Mar-13%20(3).pdf.
8. Liu LP, Wang D, Wong L, Wang YJ. (2011) Stroke and stroke care in China: Huge burden, significant workload, and a national priority. *Stroke* **42:** 3651–3654.
9. 王陇德, 刘建民, 杨弋. (2018) 中国脑卒中防治报告2017概要. 中国脑血管病杂志 **15(11):** 611–617.
10. 宇传华, 罗丽莎, 李梅. (2016) 从全球视角看中国脑卒中疾病负担的严峻性. 公共卫生与预防医学 **27(1):** 1–5.
11. 国家卫生和计划生育委员会. (2017) 2017 年中国卫生和计划生育统计年鉴. 北京: 中国协和医科大学出版社.
12. Duncan PW, Zorowitz R, Bates B, *et al.* (2005) Management of adult stroke rehabilitation care: A clinical practice guideline. *Stroke* **36(9):** e100–e143.

13. Feldman RG, Young RP, Koella WP, CIBA-GEIGY Corporation. (1980) *Spasticity: Disordered Motor Control.* Year Book Medical Publishers, Miami, FL.
14. Young RR. (1994) Spasticity: A review. *Neurology* **44(11 Suppl 9):** S12–S20.
15. Pandyan AD, Gregoric M, Barnes MP, *et al.* (2005) Spasticity: Clinical perceptions, neurological realities and meaningful measurement. *Disabil Rehabil* **27(1–2):** 2–6.
16. Robert WT, Norine CF, Norhayati H, *et al.* (2015) Evidence-based review of stroke rehabilitation. Available from: http://www.ebrsr.com/sites/default/files/documents/executive-summary-srebr_final_16ed.pdf.
17. Nair KP, Marsden J. (2014) The management of spasticity in adults. *BMJ* **349:** g4737.
18. Bates B, Choi JY, Duncan PW, *et al.* (2005) Veterans affairs/department of defense clinical practice guideline for the management of adult stroke rehabilitation care: Executive summary. *Stroke* **36(9):** 2049–2056.
19. Dietz V, Sinkjaer T. (2007) Spastic movement disorder: Impaired reflex function and altered muscle mechanics. *Lancet Neurol* **6(8):** 725–733.
20. Miller EL, Murray L, Richards L, *et al.*; American Heart Association Council on Cardiovascular Nursing and the Stroke Council. (2010) Comprehensive overview of nursing and interdisciplinary rehabilitation care of the stroke patient: A scientific statement from the American Heart Association. *Stroke* **41(10):** 2402–2448.
21. Lim SM, Yoo J, Lee E, *et al.* (2015) Acupuncture for spasticity after stroke: A systematic review and meta-analysis of randomised controlled trials. *Evid Based Complement Alternat Med* 2015: 870398.
22. Zorowitz RD, Gillard PJ, Brainin M. (2013) Poststroke spasticity: Sequelae and burden on stroke survivors and caregivers. *Neurology* **80(3 Suppl 2):** S45–S52.
23. Watkins CL, Leathley MJ, Gregson JM, *et al.* (2002) Prevalence of spasticity post stroke. *Clin Rehabil* **16(5):** 515–522.
24. Sommerfeld DK, Eek EU, Svensson AK, *et al.* (2004) Spasticity after stroke: Its occurrence and association with motor impairments and activity limitations. *Stroke* **35(1):** 134–139.
25. Kwah LK, Harvey LA, Diong JH, Herbert RD. (2012) Half of the adults who present to hospital with stroke develop at least one contracture within six months: An observational study. *J Physiother* **58(1):** 41–47.

26. Lundström E, Smits A, Borg J, Terént A. (2010) Four-fold increase in direct costs of stroke survivors with spasticity compared with stroke survivors without spasticity: The first year after the event. *Stroke* **41(2):** 319–324.
27. Bhattacharya S, Saha SP, Basu A, Das SK. (2005) A 5 years prospective study of incidence, morbidity and mortality profile of stroke in a rural community of eastern India. *J Indian Med Assoc* **103(12):** 655–659.
28. Lundström E, Terent A, Borg J. (2008) Prevalence of disabling spasticity 1 year after first-ever stroke. *Eur J Neurol* **15(6):** 533–539.
29. Brown P. (1994) Pathophysiology of spasticity. *J Neurol Neurosurg Psychiatry* **57:** 773–777.
30. Morley A, Tod A, Cramp M, Mawson S. (2013) The meaning of spasticity to people with multiple sclerosis: What can health professionals learn? *Disabil Rehabil* **35(15):** 1284–1292.
31. Esquenazi A, Mayer N. (2001) Botulinum toxin for the management of muscle overactivity and spasticity after stroke. *Curr Atheroscler Rep* **3(4):** 295–298.
32. Doan QV, Brashear A, Gillard PJ, *et al.* (2012) Relationship between disability and health-related quality of life and caregiver burden in patients with upper limb poststroke spasticity. *PM R* **4(1):** 4–10.
33. Ward AB. (2012) A literature review of the pathophysiology and onset of post-stroke spasticity. *Eur J Neurol* **19(1):** 21–27.
34. Wissel J, Schelosky LD, Scott J, *et al.* (2010) Early development of spasticity following stroke: A prospective, observational trial. *J Neurol* **257(7):** 1067–1072.
35. Urban PP, Wolf T, Uebele M, *et al.* (2010) Occurence and clinical predictors of spasticity after ischemic stroke. *Stroke* **41(9):** 2016–2020.
36. Leathley MJ, Gregson JM, Moore AP. (2004) Predicting spasticity after stroke in those surviving to 12 months. *Clin Rehabil* **18(4):** 438–443.
37. Phadke CP, Balasubramanian CK, Ismail F, Boulias C. (2013) Revisiting physiologic and psychologic triggers that increase spasticity. *Am J Phys Med Rehabil* **92(4):** 357–369.
38. Sheean G. (2002) The pathophysiology of spasticity. *Eur J Neurol* **9(Suppl 1):** 3–9.
39. Yelnik AP, Simon O, Parratte B, Gracies JM. (2010) How to clinically assess and treat muscle overactivity in spastic paresis. *J Rehabil Med* **42(9):** 801–807.

40. Malhotra S, Pandyan AD, Rosewilliam S, *et al.* (2010) Spasticity and contractures at the wrist after stroke: Time course of development and their association with functional recovery of the upper limb. *Clin Rehabil* **25(2):** 184–191.
41. Daniels J. (2009) Catatonia: Clinical aspects and neurobiological correlates. *J Neuropsychiatry Clin Neurosci* **21(4):** 371–380.
42. Bohannon RW, Smith MB. (1987) Interrater reliability of a modified Ashworth scale of muscle spasticity. *Phys Ther* **67(2):** 206–207.
43. Ashworth B. (1964) Preliminary trial of carisoprodol in multiple sclerosis. *Practitioner* **192:** 540–542.
44. Tardieu G, Shentoub S, Delarue R. (1954) Research on a technic for measurement of spasticity [Article in French]. *Rev Neurol* (Paris) **91(2):** 143–144.
45. Fosang AL, Galea MP, McCoy AT, *et al.* (2003) Measures of muscle and joint performance in the lower limb of children with cerebral palsy. *Dev Med Child Neurol* **45(10):** 664–670.
46. Mehrholz J, Wagner K, Meissner D, *et al.* (2005) Reliability of the Modified Tardieu Scale and the Modified Ashworth Scale in adult patients with severe brain injury: A comparison study. *Clin Rehabil* **19(7):** 751–759.
47. Calota A, Levin MF. (2009) Tonic stretch reflex threshold as a measure of spasticity: Implications for clinical practice. *Top Stroke Rehabil* **16(3):** 177–188.
48. Penn RD, Savoy SM, Corcos D, *et al.* (1989) Intrathecal baclofen for severe spinal spasticity. *N Engl J Med* **320(23):** 1517–1521.
49. Priebe MM, Sherwood AM, Thornby JI, *et al.* (1996) Clinical assessment of spasticity in spinal cord injury: A multidimensional problem. *Arch Phys Med Rehabil* **77(7):** 713–716.
50. Wartenberg R. (1951) Pendulousness of the legs as a diagnostic test. *Neurology* **1(1):** 18–24.
51. Biering-Sorensen F, Nielsen JB, Klinge K. (2006) Spasticity-assessment: A review. *Spinal Cord* **44(12):** 708–722.
52. Malhotra S, Pandyan AD, Day CR, *et al.* (2009) Spasticity, an impairment that is poorly defined and poorly measured. *Clin Rehabil* **23(7):** 651–658.
53. Fleuren JF, Voerman GE, Erren-Wolters CV, *et al.* (2010) Stop using the Ashworth Scale for the assessment of spasticity. *J Neurol Neurosurg Psychiatry* **81(1):** 46–52.

54. Lechner HE, Frotzler A, Eser P. (2006) Relationship between self- and clinically rated spasticity in spinal cord injury. *Arch Phys Med Rehabil* **87(1):** 15–19.
55. Hsieh JT, Wolfe DL, Miller WC, Curt A; SCIRE Research Team. (2008) Spasticity outcome measures in spinal cord injury: Psychometric properties and clinical utility. *Spinal Cord* **46(2):** 86–95.
56. 中华医学会神经病学分会神经康复学组, 中华医学会神经病学分会脑血管病学组, 卫生部脑卒中筛查与防治工程委员会办公室. 中国脑卒中康复治疗指南. *Chin J Rehabil Theory Pract* 2012; **18(4):** 18.
57. National Institute for Health and Care Excellence. (2013) Stroke rehabilitation in adults clinical guideline. Available from: https://www.nice.org.uk/guidance/cg162.
58. Stroke Foundation of New Zealand and New Zealand Guidelines Group. (2010) Clinical guidelines for stroke management. Stroke Foundation of New Zealand, Wellington. Available from: https://www.stroke.org.nz/resources/NZClinicalGuidelinesStrokeManagement2010ActiveContents.pdf.
59. Australian National Stroke Foundation. (2010) Clinical guidelines for stroke management. Available from: https://www.pedro.org.au/wp-content/uploads/CPG_stroke.pdf.
60. European Stroke Organisation (ESO) Executive Committee; ESO Writing Committee. (2008) Guidelines for management of ischaemic stroke and transient ischaemic attack. *Cerebrovasc Dis* **25(5):** 457–507.
61. Smith LN, James R, Barber M. (2010) Rehabilitation of patients with stroke: Summary of SIGN guidance. *BMJ* **340:** c2845.
62. Sheehan JL, Winzeler-Mercay U, Mudie MH. (2006) A randomised controlled pilot study to obtain the best estimate of the size of the effect of a thermoplastic resting splint on spasticity in the stroke-affected wrist and fingers. *Clin Rehabil* **20(12):** 1032–1037.
63. Bovend'Eerdt TJ, Newman M, Barker K, *et al.* (2008) The effects of stretching in spasticity: A systematic review. *Arch Phys Med Rehabil* **89(7):** 1395–1406.
64. Gustafsson L, McKenna K. (2006) A programme of static positional stretches does not reduce hemiplegic shoulder pain or maintain shoulder range of motion: A randomised controlled trial. *Clin Rehabil* **20(4):** 277–286.
65. Harvey L, de Jong I, Goehl G, Mardwedel S. (2006) Twelve weeks of nightly stretch does not reduce thumb web-space contractures in

people with a neurological condition: A randomised controlled trial. *Aust J Physiother* **52(4):** 251–258.

66. Robinson W, Smith R, Aung O, Ada L. (2008) No difference between wearing a night splint and standing on a tilt table in preventing ankle contracture early after stroke: A randomised trial. *Aust J Physiother* **54(1):** 33–38.
67. Rydwik E, Eliasson S, Akner G. (2006) The effect of exercise of the affected foot in stroke patients: A randomised controlled pilot trial. *Clin Rehabil* **20(8):** 645–655.
68. Turton AJ, Britton E. (2005) A pilot randomised controlled trial of a daily muscle stretch regime to prevent contractures in the arm after stroke. *Clin Rehabil* **19(6):** 600–612.
69. Bakhtiary AH, Fatemy E. (2008) Does electrical stimulation reduce spasticity after stroke? A randomised controlled study. *Clin Rehabil* **22(5):** 418–425.
70. Yan T, Hui-Chan CW. (2009) Transcutaneous electrical stimulation on acupuncture points improves muscle function in subjects after acute stroke: A randomised controlled trial. *J Rehabil Med* **41(5):** 312–316.
71. Hara Y, Ogawa S, Muraoka Y. (2006) Hybrid power-assisted functional electrical stimulation to improve hemiparetic upper-extremity function. *Am J Phys Med Rehabil* **85(12):** 977–985.
72. Montané E, Vallano A, Laporte JR. (2004) Oral antispastic drugs in non-progressive neurologic diseases: A systematic review. *Neurology* **63(8):** 1357–1363.
73. Simpson DM, Gracies JM, Yablon SA, *et al.*; BoNT/TZD Study Team. (2009) Botulinum neurotoxin versus tizanidine in upper limb spasticity: A placebo-controlled study. *J Neurol Neurosurg Psychiatry* **80(4):** 380–385.
74. Stamenova P, Koytchev R, Kuhn K, *et al.* (2005) A randomised, double-blind, placebo-controlled study of the efficacy and safety of tolperisone in spasticity following cerebral stroke. *Eur J Neurol* **12(6):** 453–461.
75. Bhakta BB, O'Connor RJ, Cozens JA. (2008) Associated reactions after stroke: A randomised controlled trial of the effect of botulinum toxin type A. *J Rehabil Med* **40(1):** 36–41.
76. Francis HP, Wade DT, Turner-Stokes L, *et al.* (2004) Does reducing spasticity translate into functional benefit? An exploratory meta-analysis. *J Neurol Neurosurg Psychiatry* **75(11):** 1547–1551.

77. Childers MK, Brashear A, Jozefczyk P. (2004) Dose-dependent response to intramuscular botulinum toxin type A for upper-limb spasticity in patients after a stroke. *Arch Phys Med Rehabil* **85(7):** 1063–1069.
78. Brashear A, Gordon MF, Elovic E, *et al.* (2002) Intramuscular injection of botulinum toxin for the treatment of wrist and finger spasticity after a stroke. *N Engl J Med* **347(6):** 395–400.
79. Jahangir AW, Tan HJ, Norlinah MI, *et al.* (2007) Intramuscular injection of botulinum toxin for the treatment of wrist and finger spasticity after stroke. *Med J Malaysia* **62(4):** 319–322.
80. McCrory P, Turner-Stokes L, Baguley IJ, *et al.* (2009) Botulinum toxin A for treatment of upper limb spasticity following stroke: A multi-centre randomised placebo-controlled study of the effects on quality of life and other person-centred outcomes. *J Rehabil Med* **41(7):** 536–544.
81. de Boer KS, Arwert HJ, de Groot JH, *et al.* (2008) Shoulder pain and external rotation in spastic hemiplegia do not improve by injection of botulinum toxin A into the subscapular muscle. *J Neurol Neurosurg Psychiatry* **79(5):** 581–583.
82. Kong KH, Neo JJ, Chua KS. (2007) A randomised controlled study of botulinum toxin A in the treatment of hemiplegic shoulder pain associated with spasticity. *Clin Rehabil* **21(1):** 28–35.
83. Lim JY, Koh JH, Paik NJ. (2008) Intramuscular botulinum toxin-A reduces hemiplegic shoulder pain: A randomised, double-blind, comparative study versus intraarticular triamcinolone acetonide. *Stroke* **39(1):** 126–131.
84. Marco E, Duarte E, Vila J, *et al.* (2007) Is botulinum toxin type A effective in the treatment of spastic shoulder pain in patients after stroke? A double-blind randomised clinical trial. *J Rehabil Med* **39(6):** 440–447.
85. Yelnik AP, Colle FM, Bonan IV, Vicaut E. (2007) Treatment of shoulder pain in spastic hemiplegia by reducing spasticity of the subscapular muscle: A randomised, double blind, placebo controlled study of botulinum toxin A. *J Neurol Neurosurg Psychiatry* **78(8):** 845–848.
86. Paciaroni M, Agnelli G, Micheli S, Caso V. (2007) Efficacy and safety of anticoagulant treatment in acute cardioembolic stroke: A meta-analysis of randomised controlled trials. *Stroke* **38(2):** 423–430.
87. Sampson FC, Hayward A, Evans G, *et al.* (2002) Functional benefits and cost/benefit analysis of continuous intrathecal baclofen infusion for the management of severe spasticity. *J Neurosurg* **96(6):** 1052–1057.
88. Steinbok P, O'Donnell M. (2000) Baclofen infusion for spastic cerebral palsy. *Clin Neurosurg* **47:** 440–457.

89. Kofler M, Quirbach E, Schauer R, *et al.* (2009) Limitations of intrathecal baclofen for spastic hemiparesis following stroke. *Neurorehabil Neural Repair* **23(1):** 26–31.
90. Liu X, Bao C, Dong G. (2014) Using acupoint-to-acupoint penetrative needling to treat post-stroke spastic paralysis: A clinical progress review. *J Tradit Chin Med* **34(5):** 609–615.
91. Vados L, Ferreira A, Zhao S, *et al.* (2015) Effectiveness of acupuncture combined with rehabilitation for treatment of acute or subacute stroke: A systematic review. *Acupunct Med* **33(3):** 180–187.
92. Lim SM, Yoo J, Lee E, *et al.* (2015) Acupuncture for spasticity after stroke: A systematic review and meta-analysis of randomised controlled trials. *Evid Based Complement Alternat Med* **2015:** 870398.
93. 陈紫薇, 谭子虎, 芍药甘草汤治疗中风后痉挛性偏瘫的系统评价. (2016) 云南中医中药杂志 **37(2):** 23–26.
94. 范江华, 黄永, 王开龙, 马甜, 雷龙鸣. (2016) 从循证医学角度分析推拿治疗中风后痉挛性偏瘫的疗效. 中国中医基础医学杂志 **22(2):** 242–248.
95. 王开龙, 黄永, 范江华. (2016) 推拿治疗脑卒中痉挛状态的 meta 分析. 中国民族民间医药 **25(3):** 24–29.

2

Post-stroke Spasticity in Chinese Medicine

OVERVIEW

In Chinese medicine, post-stroke spasticity is considered a condition with deficiency in the root (本虚) and excess in the superficiality (标实), and closely related to the function of Liver and Kidney organs, *qi* 气 and Blood. This chapter provides an overview of the aetiology, pathogenesis, syndrome differentiation and related therapies of post-stroke spasticity in current Chinese medicine textbooks, clinical guidelines and related monographs.

Introduction

Hemiplegia, as one of the major complications of stroke, can be classified into flaccid paralysis and spastic paralysis. Flaccid paralysis occurs in the initial stage of stroke and then it may develop into the spastic type in two weeks, which may last for a long period of time. According to the traditional Chinese medicine (CM) theory, post-stroke spasticity can be categorised as 'tendon disease 筋病' and 'spastic syndrome 痉证'. The term '*jing luan* 痉挛 (spasticity)' was firstly recorded in the ancient book *Ling Shu* (灵枢 – 刺节真邪) as the name of the syndrome. It was described in *Su Wen* (素问 – 长刺节论篇) that 'when tendons are diseased, spasticity and joint pain occur, causing movement difficulties. This is called tendon impediment (*Bi* syndrome 痹证)' (病在筋, 筋挛节痛, 不可以行, 名曰筋痹). This description indicates that the tendon contracture will lead to difficult movement of limbs. The *yin* and *yang* 阴阳 theory of CM pointed out that the fundamental reason of post-stroke spasticity is the *yin-yang* imbalance. For instance, it was recorded in the book *Nan Jing* (难经) that 'When the *yin*-heel vessel is diseased, the *yin* 阴 part of muscles will be tense and the *yang* 阳 part of muscles will be relaxed. While when the *yang*-heel vessel is diseased, the *yang* 阳 part of muscles will be tense and the *yin* 阴 part of muscles will be relaxed.' (阴跷为病, 阳缓而阴急; 阳跷为病, 阴缓而阳急).

Aetiology and Pathogenesis

Spasticity, as one of the major complications of stroke, is considered as a condition with deficiency in the root (本虚) and excess in the superficiality (标实), and closely related to the function of Liver and Kidney organs, *qi* 气 and Blood.

The characteristics of the symptoms suggest that spasticity is caused fundamentally by *yin* 阴 deficiency of the Liver and Kidney resulting in *qi* 气 and Blood deficiency, which causes the failure of nourishing the tendons (this is considered as the deficiency in the root 本虚), and therefore limb stiffness and contracture occurs (this is considered as the excess in the superficiality 标实).

Syndrome Differentiation and Treatments

Post-stroke spasticity is considered to originate from the combination of deficiency (*yin* 阴, Kidney, Liver and Blood), Wind, Blood stasis, and Phlegm stagnation. When stroke happens, the vital *qi* 气 is damaged and pathogenesis is lingering, patients' extremities undergo lack of nourishing and hence spasticity will gradually occur. Therefore, the treatment principle for post-stroke spasticity is to tonify the Liver and Kidney, nourish *qi* 气 and Blood, soften the tendons, and smooth meridians and collaterals. Historically, in order to enhance the tonifying effects, some ingredients that originated from animals and bugs may be considered.

Other than Chinese herbal medicine (CHM), acupuncture, massage and other CM rehabilitation therapies, or their combinations, can also be applied for the management of post-stroke spasticity as indicated below. In current clinical guidelines and textbooks, the syndrome differentiation and accompanying treatments are not discussed in detail. The treatment methods listed below originated and are modified from the contents of the monograph 神经系统疾病功能障碍中西医康复.[1]

Oral Chinese Herbal Medicine

Main symptoms: Paralysis, spasticity or even stiffness and deformation of limb(s), difficult movement (often accompanied with numbness), slightly red tongue with thin and white (or with scanty) coating, fine and string-like pulse (or deep and fine pulse).[1]

Treatment principle: Nourishing *qi* 气 and Blood 益气血, tonifying the Liver and Kidney 补肝肾, and unblocking meridians 通经脉.[1]

Formula: Modified *Bu yang huan wu tang* 补阳还五汤 in combination with *Di huang yin zi* 地黄饮子.[1]

Ingredients: *Huang qi* 黄芪, *dang gui* 当归, *tao ren* 桃仁, *hong hua* 红花, *huai niu xi* 怀牛膝, *shu di huang* 熟地黄, *shan yu rou* 山萸肉, *mai dong* 麦冬, *shi hu* 石斛, *ba ji tian* 巴戟天, *rou cong rong* 肉苁蓉, *chang pu* 菖蒲, *fu ling* 茯苓, *ji xue teng* 鸡血藤, *mu gua* 木瓜, *bai shao* 白芍 and *zhi gan cao* 炙甘草.[1]

Modification according to syndrome differentiation:[1]

- For patients with syndrome of phlegm stagnation, add *fa ban xia* 法半夏, *bai zhu* 白术 and *dan nan xing* 胆南星;
- For patients with syndrome of *yin* 阴 deficiency and internal Wind, add *wu gong* 蜈蚣, *quan xie* 全蝎 and *wu shao she* 乌梢蛇;
- For patients with syndrome of *yang* 阳 deficiency and cold limbs, add *zhi fu zi* 制附子 and *gui zhi* 桂枝.

Main actions of herbs: *Huang qi* 黄芪 should be used in a relatively large dose to tonify *qi* 气; *dang gui* 当归, *tao ren* 桃仁, *hong hua* 红花 and *huai niu xi* 怀牛膝 together work to tonify Blood and remove Blood stasis; *shu di huang* 熟地黄 and *shan yu rou* 山萸肉 will tonify

Kidney and Essence; *mai dong* 麦冬 and *shi hu* 石斛 work to tonify *yin* 阴; *ba ji tian* 巴戟天 and *rou cong rong* 肉苁蓉 will warm and tonify Kidney *yang* 阳; *chang pu* 菖蒲 and *fu ling* 茯苓 will remove Phlegm and open orifices; *ji xue teng* 鸡血藤, *mu gua* 木瓜, *bai shao* 白芍 and *zhi gan cao* 炙甘草 will tonify Blood, soften tendons and unblock meridians.

Topical Chinese Herbal Medicine

Chinese herbal medicine can be topically applied through paste, and steaming and bathing therapy, as detailed below:

Chinese Herbal Medicine Paste Topical Application

Ingredients: *Dang gui* 当归, *chuang xiong* 川芎, *bing pian* 冰片, *chuan niu xi* 川牛膝, *tou gu cao* 透骨草, *wei ling xian* 威灵仙, *hong hua* 红花, *fang feng* 防风, *ai ye* 艾叶, *gui zhi* 桂枝 and *zhe chong* 蟅虫.[2]

Method: Use the above ingredients in the same quantities and grind into a rough powder, then mix with vinegar, liquor and wood oil to make a paste.[2] Apply a proper amount of the paste on acupuncture points of ST36 *Zusanli* 足三里, GB20 *Fengchi* 风池, LI10 *Shousanli* 手三里, LI11 *Quchi* 曲池 and LI15 *Jianyu* 肩髃 of the diseased side, once a day, 20–30 minutes each time, continually for 30 days as a treatment course.[2]

Chinese Herbal Medicine Steaming Therapy and Bathing Therapy

CHM formula: *Fu fang tong luo ye* 复方通络液.

Ingredients: *Hong hua* 红花, *chuan wu* 川乌, *cao wu* 草乌, *dang gui* 当归, *chuang xiong* 川芎 and *sang zhi* 桑枝.[3]

Method: Make a 1000–2000 mL decoction using the above ingredients, and apply steaming followed by bathing therapies using the decoction on the affected side.[3]

Chinese Herbal Medicine Steaming Therapy

CHM formula: *Kang jing luan fang* 抗痉挛方.

Ingredients: *Bai shao* 白芍, *wang jiang nan* 望江南, *shen jin cao* 伸筋草, *mu gua* 木瓜, *sang zhi* 桑枝, *hong hua* 红花, *dang gui* 当归, *ru xiang* 乳香 and *mo yao* 没药.[2]

Method: Soak the above ingredients in water for 30 minutes, then make the decoction using a pot which is specially designed for CHM steaming therapy. The CHM steam will be transferred to a therapeutic cabin, in which the temperature is pre-set to 37℃. Patients then receive steaming therapy in the cabin for 20 minutes.[2]

Main actions of herbs: All these herbs used topically, either as topically applied CHM paste or steaming/bathing therapy, share similar functions as those used orally. For example, *hong hua* 红花, *dang gui* 当归, *chuang xiong* 川芎 and *niu xi* 牛膝 work together to tonify Blood and remove Blood stasis; *chuan wu* 川乌, *cao wu* 草乌, *ru xiang* 乳香 and *mo yao* 没药 remove Blood stasis and relieve pain; *wei ling xian* 威灵仙, *gui zhi* 桂枝, *sang zhi* 桑枝, *tou gu cao* 透骨草 and *shen jin cao* 伸筋草 unblock meridians and nourish tendons and muscles; and *mu gua* 木瓜 softens tendons and reduce spasticity.

Acupuncture Therapy

Acupuncture therapy should be applied taking syndrome differentiation into consideration, with more focus placed on affected muscles. It should be pointed out that acupuncture stimulation can be applied on antagonistic muscles but avoid spastic muscles. Apply mild stimulation on the antagonistic muscles which are associated with those spastic muscles, so that the antagonistic muscles are activated, and the spastic muscles are inhibited.[4] Points can be selected from the following list based on the affected muscles:

- Spasticity of the upper limb flexor muscle: TE13 *Naohui* 臑会, SI9 *Jianzhen* 肩贞, TE10 *Tianjing* 天井, LI10 *Shousanli* 手三里, TE5

Waiguan 外关, TE4 *Yangchi* 阳池 and TE3 *Zhongzhu* 中渚 on the diseased side;
- Spasticity of the upper limb extensor muscle: LI11 *Quchi* 曲池, PC6 *Neiguan* 内关 and PC5 *Jianshi* 间使 on the diseased side;
- Spasticity of the lower limb extensor muscle: BL37 *Yinmen* 殷门, BL40 *Weizhong* 委中, BL39 *Weiyang* 委阳, BL57 *Chengshan* 承山, GB34 *Yanglingquan* 阳陵泉 and KI6 *Zhaohai* 照海 on the diseased side;
- Spasticity of the lower limb flexor muscle: ST32 *Futu* 伏兔, ST33 *Yinshi* 阴市, ST34 *Liangqiu* 梁丘, ST40 *Fenglong* 丰隆 and ST37 *Shangjuxu* 上巨虚 on the diseased side.

Warm Needling

Warm needling technique is a treatment combining acupuncture and moxibustion.[4]

Point selection based on the affected muscles is shown below:

- Upper limb of affected side: LU5 *Chize* 尺泽, LI11 *Quchi* 曲池, LI10 *Shousanli* 手三里, PC6 *Neiguan* 内关 and LI4 *Hegu* 合谷;
- Lower limb of the affected side: GB30 *Huantiao* 环跳, GB31 *Fengshi* 风市, SP10 *Xuehai* 血海, GB34 *Yanglingquan* 阳陵泉, GB40 *Qiuxu* 丘墟 and LR3 *Taichong* 太冲.

Method: Firstly, needling certain acupuncture points with twirling and rotating needles for neutral supplementation and draining can be used. Then apply moxibustion cones on top of the needle handles. Three *Zhuang* 壮 of moxibustion cones will be applied on each needle/point, or up to the patient's level of tolerance. This treatment is performed once a day, for a total of 30 days.[4]

***Tuina* 推拿 Therapy**

Point selection:

- Upper limb: GB21 *Jianjing* 肩井, LI14 *Binao* 臂臑, LI11 *Quchi* 曲池, TE5 *Waiguan* 外关 and LI4 *Hegu* 合谷;

- Lower limb: GB34 *Yanglingquan* 阳陵泉, GB31 *Fengshi* 风市, EX-LE5 *Xiyan* 膝眼, ST41 *Jiexi* 解溪, GB40 *Qiuxu* 丘墟 and LR3 *Taichong* 太冲.

Manual manipulation: Gently and slowly move the joint, with appropriate rhythm. Point pressing 点按, *qi*-concentrated single-finger manipulation 一指禅, and finger vibrating 指振法 are mostly applied. For antagonistic muscles, strong and more intense manipulation techniques such as rolling 滚法, point-pressing 点按 and flicking 弹拨 for restoring the muscle strength can be utilised.[5]

Prevention and Lifestyle Adjustment

For patients who have severe spasticity, staying in bed and avoiding physical activities is preferable. It is important to avoid stretching or pressing the affected limbs by force in case the strongly increased muscle tone will cause bone fractures.

In terms of prevention and maintenance, patients and their families or carers should be aware that some factors may aggravate

Table 2.1 Summary of Chinese Medicine Therapies

Therapies	Herbs/Acupuncture Points	Treatment Methods
Oral CHM	*Bu yang huan wu tang* 补阳还五汤 in combination with *Di huang yin zi* 地黄饮子.	—
CHM: Paste topical application	*Dang gui* 当归, *chuang xiong* 川芎, *bing pian* 冰片, *chuan niu xi* 川牛膝, *tou gu cao* 透骨草, *wei ling xian* 威灵仙, *hong hua* 红花, *fang feng* 防风, *ai ye* 艾叶, *gui zhi* 桂枝 and *zhe chong* 蛰虫.	Grind these herbs into a rough powder and mix with vinegar, liquor and wood oil to make a paste. Apply this CHM paste on acupuncture points of ST36 *Zusanli* 足三里, GB20 *Fengchi* 风池, LI10 *Shousanli* 手三里, LI11 *Quchi* 曲池 and LI15 *Jianyu* 肩髃 of the affected side.

(*Continued*)

Table 2.1 (*Continued*)

Therapies	Herbs/Acupuncture Points	Treatment Methods
CHM: Steaming therapy and bathing therapy	*Fu fang tong luo ye* 复方通络液.	Make 1000–2000 mL decoction using these herbs; apply steaming followed by bathing therapies using the decoction on the affected side.
CHM: Steaming therapy	*Kang jing luan fang* 抗痉挛方.	Make decoction using these herbs, then transfer the CHM steam to a specific therapeutic cabin for patients to receive steaming therapy.
Acupuncture	• Upper limb flexor muscle: TE13 *Naohui* 臑会, SI9 *Jianzhen* 肩贞, TE10 *Tianjing* 天井, LI10 *Shousanli* 手三里, TE5 *Waiguan* 外关, TE4 *Yangchi* 阳池 and TE3 *Zhongzhu* 中渚 on the diseased side; • Upper limb extensor muscle: LI11 *Quchi* 曲池, PC6 *Neiguan* 内关 and PC5 *Jianshi* 间使 on the diseased side; • Lower limb extensor muscle: BL37 *Yinmen* 殷门, BL40 *Weizhong* 委中, BL39 *Weiyang* 委阳, BL57 *Chengshan* 承山, GB34 *Yanglingquan* 阳陵泉 and KI6 *Zhaohai* 照海 on the diseased side; • Lower limb flexor muscle: ST32 *Futu* 伏兔, ST33 *Yinshi* 阴市, ST34 *Liangqiu* 梁丘, ST40 *Fenglong* 丰隆 and ST37 *Shangjuxu* 上巨虚 on the diseased side.	Acupuncture stimulation can be applied on antagonistic muscles but avoid spastic muscles. Apply mild stimulation on the antagonistic muscles which are associated with those spastic muscles, so that the antagonistic muscles are activated, and the spastic muscles are inhibited.

(*Continued*)

Table 2.1 (*Continued*)

Therapies	Herbs/Acupuncture Points	Treatment Methods
Warm needling	• Upper limb of affected side: LU5 *Chize* 尺泽, LI11 *Quchi* 曲池, LI10 *Shousanli* 手三里, PC6 *Neiguan* 内关 and LI4 *Hegu* 合谷; • Lower limb of the affected side: GB30 *Huantiao* 环跳, GB31 *Fengshi* 风市, SP10 *Xuehai* 血海, GB34 *Yanglingquan* 阳陵泉, GB40 *Qiuxu* 丘墟 and LR3 *Taichong* 太冲.	Needling certain acupuncture points with twirling and rotating needles for neutral supplementation and draining can be used. Then apply moxibustion cones on top of the needle handles.
Tuina 推拿 therapy	• Upper limb: GB21 *Jianjing* 肩井, LI14 *Binao* 臂臑, LI11 *Quchi* 曲池, TE5 *Waiguan* 外关 and LI4 *Hegu* 合谷; • Lower limb: GB34 *Yanglingquan* 阳陵泉, GB31 *Fengshi* 风市, EX-LE5 *Xiyan* 膝眼, ST41 *Jiexi* 解溪, GB40 *Qiuxu* 丘墟 and LR3 *Taichong* 太冲.	Mainly apply mild stimulation with point pressing 点按, *qi*-concentrated single-finger manipulation 一指禅 and finger vibrating 指振法. Strong and more intense manipulation techniques can be used on antagonistic muscles.

Abbreviations: CHM — Chinese herbal medicine.

spasticity, such as pressure sores, bone fractures, skin infections, inappropriate position, anxiety and constipation. Such factors should be avoided as much as possible in stroke patients' daily life. Gentle exercise individually designed according to the patient's conditions are encouraged.

In addition, some CM therapies, which are not commonly practised in countries or areas outside of China, have also been recommended, e.g. *Gua sha* 刮痧 (scraping therapy). These are not discussed in this chapter.

References

1. 陈红霞. (2016) 神经系统疾病功能障碍中西医康复. 北京: 人民卫生出版社.
2. 陈红霞. (2009) 中风病的中西医结合康复治疗. 北京: 人民卫生出版社.
3. 中华中医药学会. (2008) 中医内科常见病诊疗指南·西医疾病部分. 北京: 中国中医药出版社.
4. 王永炎, 谢雁鸣. (2010) 实用中风病康复学. 北京: 人民卫生出版社.
5. 中国中医科学院. (2011) 中医循证临床实践指南 — 中医内科. 北京: 中国中医药出版社.

3

Classical Chinese Medicine Literature

OVERVIEW

Classical Chinese medicine literature provides a rich source of information for prevention and management of diseases. There may be some treatments used in contemporary practice that date back to classical literature, including current treatments for post-stroke spasticity. This chapter describes the findings of a systematic search of the *Zhong Hua Yi Dian* 中华医典, based on a selection of search terms identified from classical dictionaries and texts. Search of the *Zhong Hua Yi Dian* 中华医典 located over 1,100 citations which were analysed to identify the common formulas, herbs and acupuncture points used to treat symptoms 'possibly' or 'likely' corresponding to post-stroke spasticity.

Introduction

Chinese medicine therapies have been practised for a long time. Generally it is thought that acupuncture originated in ancient China during the late Spring and Autumn (770–476 BC) or early Warring States (474–221 BC) periods,[1,2] and the practice of Chinese herbal medicine (CHM) was first recorded in the oldest surviving book on materia medica, *Shen Nong Ben Cao Jing* 神农本草经, in the Western Han dynasty (206 BC–24 AD).[3,4] Since then, a large amount of literature has accumulated along with the thousands of years of Chinese medicine (CM) clinical practice. It is likely that there has been some descriptions recorded in the vast classical literature referring to the symptoms similar to stroke and post-stroke complications. In order to systematically summarise such information from classical CM literature, the digitalised collections *Zhong Hua Yi Dian* (ZHYD) 中华医典

CD-ROM — a collection of more than 1,000 medical books of the classical CM literature, was searched. *Zhong Hua Yi Dian* 中华医典 is currently the largest collection of the classical and pre-modern CM literature.[3–5]

Stroke is a serious clinical condition which occurs when a part of the brain is damaged due to lack of blood supply. The symptoms of stroke vary greatly according to the function of the affected part of the brain. According to the ancient CM concept, *feng* 风 (Wind) was described as 'travel fast and change greatly 善行而数变'. Therefore, based on the observation of clinical symptoms, stroke was named as *zhong feng* 中风, which refers to 'a sudden Wind attack'. However, the term *zhong feng* 中风 might also have been used to describe other clinical conditions. In order to systematically evaluate the CM classical literature to identify likely therapies for post-stroke spasticity, it should be taken into consideration that these therapies may have been introduced under a variety of disease names or descriptions of symptoms.

Search Terms

Due to the nature of language development over time, there have additional terms to *zhong feng* 中风, which also referred to this clinical condition. Recent research suggested that, since the era of *Huang Di Nei Jing* 黄帝内经 until the Qing dynasty (before 1911), there have been more than 30 names used in different books corresponding to the condition of stroke; these include *pian ku* 偏枯, *pian feng* 偏风, *tan huan* 瘫缓, *tan huan* 瘫痪, *zuo tan* 左瘫, *you huan* 右痪, *wei tui feng* 猥腿风, *da jue* 大厥, *jian jue* 煎厥, *bo jue* 薄厥, *pu ji* 仆击, *cu zhong* 卒中, *zhong feng* 中风, *fei feng* 肺风, *xin feng* 心风, *gan feng* 肝风, *pi feng* 脾风, *shen feng* 肾风, *fei zhong feng* 肺中风, *xin zhong feng* 心中风, *gan zhong feng* 肝中风, *pi zhong feng* 脾中风, *shen zhong feng* 肾中风, *nao feng* 脑风, *mu feng* 目风, *shou feng* 首风, *nei feng* 内风, *fei feng* 痱风, *feng qi* 风气, *wu fei* 瘖痱, *bao wu* 暴瘖, *feng yi* 风懿, *feng bi* 风痹, *wei feng* 微风, *lou feng* 漏风 and *lao feng* 劳风.[6] Therefore, it is necessary to identify the most relevant terms for accurately locating potential treatments of post-stroke spasticity from the large amount of classical literature.

Firstly, prior to the comprehensive search conducted using the ZHYD 中华医典 CD-ROM, search terms were identified through a systematic screening process. Since post-stroke spasticity was not an independent disease in history, we conducted a search in classical literature using terms of overall stroke and post-stroke motor and functional impairment. By reviewing five CM books or clinical guidelines[7–11] and 20 journal articles or thesis[12–31] on stroke classical terminology, a total of 61 terms were extracted and used in trial searches in the ZHYD. All 61 terms were used for a preliminary test search and the search yielded a total of over 46,000 search results.

Through discussion of the preliminary results with clinical experts, 12 search terms were finally selected as most relevant to stroke and post-stroke complications. These were *Zhong feng* 中风, *zhong jing* 中经, *zhong zang* 中脏, *bo jue* 薄厥, *cu zhong* (1) 猝中, *cu zhong* (2) 卒中, *feng fei* 风痱, *pian feng* 偏风, *pian ku* 偏枯, *tan huan* 瘫痪, *ban shen bu sui* (1) 半身不遂 and *ban shen bu sui* (2) 半身不随 (Table 3.1). Other terms were not considered

Table 3.1 Terms Used to Identify Classical Literature Citations

Search Terms in Pinyin	Search Terms in Chinese	English Translation
Zhong feng	中风	Sudden Wind attack
Zhong jing	中经	Hemiplegia-type dysfunction post-Wind attack
Zhong zang	中脏	Visceral stroke
Bo jue	薄厥	Flopping syncope
Cu zhong (1)	猝中	Sudden Wind attack
Cu zhong (2)	卒中	Sudden Wind attack
Feng fei	风痱	Sudden Wind attack
Pian feng	偏风	Hemiplegia-type Wind attack
Pian ku	偏枯	Hemiplegia-type dysfunction
Tan huan	瘫痪	Paralysis
Ban shen bu sui (1)	半身不遂	Hemiplegia
Ban shen bu sui (2)	半身不随	Hemiplegia

for use in our final search since they were deemed not highly relevant to stroke or brought duplicated descriptions with other more promising terms.

Procedures for Search, Data Coding and Data Analysis

The procedure for searching the ZHYD, screening and analysis is presented in Fig. 3.1. Each of the 12 search terms was entered into the ZHYD search fields. The initial search yielded a total of 29,125 search results, and 27,460 remained for screening after removing duplicates. Results of each search term were downloaded and entered into spreadsheets, with a distinct passage of text containing the specific description of symptoms and/or treatments considered as one citation for further analysis. Where the same information was identified by different search terms, only one citation was kept in the dataset but labelled with multiple search terms. All relevant citations were reviewed for exclusions from further analyses if they were:

- Not related to stroke;
- Of paediatric diseases;

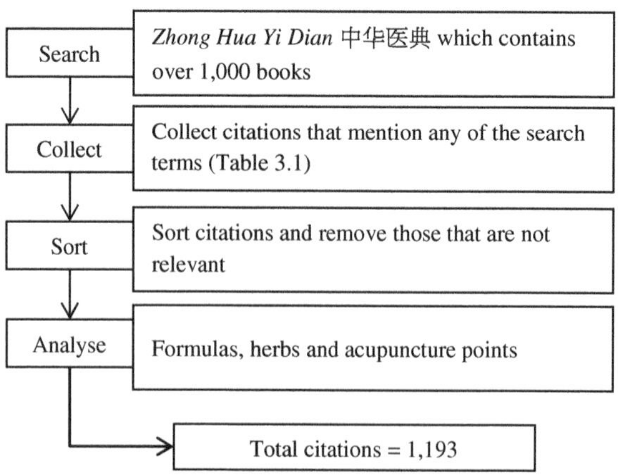

Fig. 3.1 Classical literature citations.

- Related to stroke but not about motor and functional impairment;
- Related to post-stroke motor and functional impairment but mentioning symptoms likely referring to hypomyotonia;
- Not containing information of treatment.

The final dataset (*n* = 1,193) following exclusion was limited to the citations considered potentially referring to 'possibly related to post-stroke spasticity', with description of CM treatments (CHM, acupuncture and related therapies, or other CM therapies). If one citation contained multiple treatments (e.g. multiple CHM formulas), they were separated for calculation of formulas, herbs or acupuncture points. For the pharmacopeia entries, only those that provided a detailed description of the condition or information about treatment were included for further analyses. This procedure is shown in Fig. 3.1.

Furthermore, a more focused screening was conducted to identify the treatments 'most likely related to post-stroke spasticity'. Citations that described the spasticity-like symptoms were included in this pool. Examples of the spasticity-like symptoms are as follows: arm and leg muscular contracture (*shou zu ju luan* 手足拘挛), contracture or limb spasm (*ju ji* 拘急), spasm of muscle (*jin luan* 筋挛), spasm and contracture (*luan suo* 挛缩, *luan bi* 挛躄), muscle spasm and contracture (*jin mai luan ji* 筋脉挛急, *jin ji* 筋急, *chi cong* 瘛疭), muscle contracture and stiffness of limbs (*ju luan qu shen bu de* 拘挛屈伸不得), and muscle contracture and atrophy after wind attack (*jiu feng ku zhi* 久风枯挚).

Lastly, all data were presented for the frequencies of identified formulas, herbs and acupuncture points within two levels: (1) citations that were 'possibly' related to post-stroke spasticity, and (2) citations that were 'most likely' related to post-stroke spasticity.

Search Results

The initial search using the 12 search terms obtained a total of 27,460 instants (hits) for further screening and analyses; the results are shown in Table 3.2. The search term which produced

Table 3.2 Hit Frequencies by Search Term

Pinyin	Chinese Characters	Hit Frequency (*n*, %)
Zhong feng	中风	19,150 (69.7)
Tan huan	瘫痪	1,532 (5.6)
Pian ku	偏枯	1,521 (5.5)
Ban shen bu sui (1)	半身不遂	1,380 (5.0)
Cu zhong (2)	卒中	1,261 (4.6)
Pian feng	偏风	907 (3.3)
Zhong zang	中脏	611 (2.2)
Zhong jing	中经	435 (1.6)
Bo jue	薄厥	208 (0.8)
Cu zhong (1)	猝中	206 (0.8)
Feng fei	风痱	204 (0.7)
Ban shen bu sui (2)	半身不随	45 (0.2)
Total		27,460 (100)

the highest number of hits was *zhong feng* 中风 (19,150 hits, 69.7%). All other search terms were identified in less than 6% of all hits (Table 3.2).

Citations Included for Analyses

After removal of exclusions, a total of 1,193 citations were included as 'possibly related to post-stroke spasticity'. Among them, 1,028 citations focused on CHM treatments, and 165 citations described some acupuncture-related therapies. Forty-eight citations reported clinical case reports. Among all these included citations, 264 citations were further judged as 'most likely related to post-stroke spasticity' since they specified symptoms of muscle contracture and stiffness or likely hypermyotonia.

Definitions of the Condition and Aetiology

In CM classical literature, post-stroke spasticity was not considered as an independent clinical condition; it was stated in the discussions of stroke (*zhong feng* 中风) as one of the symptoms. The definition of stroke (*zhong feng* 中风) in ancient China was similar to that in the modern concept, since it was based on the observation of clinical symptoms. In particular, medical literature in the Ming and Qing dynasty recorded detailed symptoms caused by *zhong feng* 中风. Examples are given below:

1. 'Mr. Lou said that *zhong feng* 中风 was a common name of the disease which presents as a sudden fall, facial paralysis, hemiplegia, stiff tongue with aphasia, and mouth opened cannot close. However, symptoms may vary from person to person. Since it often presents as a sudden fall, it used to be called as *ji pu* 击仆 or *cu zhong* 卒中 because it was considered similar to a sudden Wind attack. For the symptoms of facial paralysis and hemiplegia, it used to be called *pian ku* 偏枯 or *zuo tan you huan* 左瘫右痪' (*Ji Yang Gang Mu* 济阳纲目•论风分在腑在脏在经浅深之异, c. 1626);
2. 'A person suddenly fell and the body became stiff, may present the symptoms of hemiplegia, or bilateral limbs paralysis, or unconsciousness. This person may, or may not, die. It is called *zhong feng* 中风' (*Yi Jing Su Hui Ji* 医经溯洄集•中风辨, c. 1368);
3. '*Zhong feng* 中风 presents as a sudden fall, unconsciousness, large amount of sputum accumulated in the throat with snoring sound. The patient may present facial paralysis, bilateral limbs paralysis or hemiplegia, mouth closed with lockjaw, stiff tongue, and aphasia' (*Yi Bian* 医碥•中风, c. 1751).

In addition to the description of symptoms, the aetiology of *zhong feng* 中风 had also been discussed continually in history. *Zhong feng* 中风 was initially thought to be caused by an external pathogen, and then developed to become internal factors. For example, in early times, *zhong feng* 中风 was believed to be caused by external wind attack combining with internal *qi* 气 deficiency (e.g. *pian ku* 偏枯 is caused by deficiency of one side of the body. When there is deficiency of defending *qi* 气, an external pathogen will attack this side of body and cause disease (*Ling Shu* 灵枢•刺节真邪)); meanwhile, the patient's constitution was also noted to be a potential risk factor of *zhong feng* 中风 (*pian ku* 偏枯 and some other conditions could be caused by overweight/obesity, it is also considered as disease caused by long-term intake of fatty food (*Su Wen* 素问•通评虚实论)).

In the Yuan and Ming dynasty, the internal factors including internal deficiency, and Phlegm and Heat were considered to be the main causalities of *zhong feng* 中风. For instance:

- Internal deficiency 内虚

'*Zhong feng* 中风 is not caused by an external pathogen. In fact, it is caused by internal factors. One who is over 40 years old, his *qi* 气 starts to get less and less sufficient; if he also gets emotions pent-up, the deficient *qi* 气 will be further damaged. Hence people in this age commonly suffer from the condition of *zhong feng* 中风 but younger people are less likely to get this disease. In particular, people who are overweight are more likely to be affected by this disease because being overweight will further damage his *qi* 气' (*Yi Xue Fa Ming* 医学发明•中风有三, c. 1315).

'A condition named *fei feng* 非风, it is commonly called as *zhong feng* 中风. Symptoms include sudden falling often accompanied by unconsciousness. This is caused by long-term internal deficiency rather than external Wind-cold invasion' (*Jing Yue Quan Shu* 景岳全书•非风, c. 1624).

- Internal Phlegm 痰蕴

'People live in the east-south may suffer from a type of "Wind" disease. In fact, it is not real external Wind invasion. The real reason is middle-*jiao* 焦 dampness causing Phlegm, then Heat will be generated from the Phlegm and disturbing *qi* 气, therefore internal Wind occurred' (*Dan Xi Xin Fa* 丹溪心法•论中风, c. 1347).

'Hemiplegia, most of the cases were caused by Phlegm. The left side of the body is paralysed, and it is due to dead Blood or insufficient Blood. Treatment: can consider *Si wu tang* 四物汤 plus *tao ren* 桃仁, *hong hua* 红花, *zhu li* 竹沥, and ginger juice 姜汁. While if the right side of the body is paralysed, it is caused by Phlegm and *qi* 气 deficiency, in treatment one may consider *Er chen tang* 二陈汤 plus *Si jun zi tang* 四君子汤 adding *zhu li* 竹沥, mixed with ginger juice 姜汁' (*Dan Xi Xin Fa* 丹溪心法•论中风, c. 1347).

- Internal Heat 内热

'Due to lack of resting, there is internal Heat and Fire growing. If such Heat is out of control, there will be *yin* 阴 deficiency and excess *yang* 阳 uprising. The deficient Heat will cause *qi* 气 being stagnated and therefore *shen* 神 became unclear, leading to sudden falling and unconsciousness' (*He Jian Liu Shu* 河间六书•素问玄机原病式, Ming dynasty).

In the Qing dynasty, internal Wind of Liver *yang* 阳 uprising was thought to be the real reason of *zhong feng* 中风. This is consistent with current understanding of the stroke aetiology:

'For a person who has Blood and Essences deficiency, water is not sufficient to nourish wood, hence liver *yang* uprising causes internal Wind' (*Lin Zheng Zhi Nan* 临证指南•中风, c. 1746).

'Doctor Hua recorded that Doctor Ye created the name of "internal Wind" 内风, which is caused by unstable *yang qi* 阳气 in the body. Liver is known as both the Wood organ and the Wind organ, if Water is insufficient, the Wood will not be nourished. Therefore the Liver *yang* 阳 will upraise and cause internal Wind. In this case, the treatment should consider nourishing *yin* 阴 and eliminating Wind...' (*Lin Zheng Zhi Nan Yi An* 临证指南医案•中风, c. 1746).

Chinese Herbal Medicine

A total of 1,028 citations included 'possible post-stroke spasticity' and introduced CHM treatments. They were found in 226 books. The books with the largest number of citations were *Pu Ji Fang* 普济方 (c. 1406) ($n = 105$), *Sheng Ji Zong Lu* 圣济总录 (c. 1117) ($n = 89$), *Tai Ping Sheng Hui Fang* 太平圣惠方 (c. 992) ($n = 72$), *Ji Yang Gang Mu* 济阳纲目 (c. 1626) ($n = 49$), *Qi Xiao Liang Fang* 奇效良方 (c. 1470) ($n = 27$), *Gu Jin Yi Tong Da Quan* 古今医统大全 (c. 1556) ($n = 19$), *Wai Tai Mi Yao* 外台秘要 (c. 752) ($n = 18$), *Bei Ji Qian Jin Yao Fang* 备急千金要方 (c. 652) ($n = 16$), *Tai Ping Hui Min He Ji Ju Fang* 太平惠民和剂局方 (c. 1151) ($n = 15$) and *Yi Xue Gang Mu* 医学纲目 (c. 1565) ($n = 14$).

Frequency of Treatment Citations by Dynasty

Almost two thirds (66.3%) of the 'possible post-stroke spasticity' citations were identified from books of the Ming dynasty (c. 1369–1644) and Qing dynasty (c. 1645–1911) (Table 3.3). Two citations were from books without a known publishing year, and two citations were from a CHM book published in Japan (c. 1780).

The earliest citation identified by the search term *zhong feng* 中风 containing three treatments was retrieved from *Hua Tuo Shen Fang* 华佗神方 (Han dynasty). The most recent citations were from the book named *Zhong Feng Jiao Quan* 中风斠诠 (c. 1917) and were identified by three search terms: *zhong feng* 中风, *ban shen bu sui* 半身不遂 and *pian feng* 偏风.

The CHM treatments described in all 'possible post-stroke spasticity' citations were analysed for frequency of formula names and herb ingredients. If ingredients were not specified in the included citation, the book where this citation was found was searched to identify other instances of the same formula for its ingredients. If identified, these ingredients were used for further analysis of herb frequencies.

Table 3.3 Dynastic Distribution of Chinese Herbal Medicine Treatment Citations

Dynasty	No. of Treatment Citations
Before Tang dynasty (before 618)	4
Tang and 5 dynasties (618–960)	44
Song and Jin dynasties (961–1271)	240
Yuan dynasty (1272–1368)	31
Ming dynasty (1369–1644)	416
Qing dynasty (1645–1911)	266
Min Guo/Republic of China (1912–1949)	23
Others	2 unknown, 2 Japan*
Total	**1,028**

*Chinese medicine books published in Japan.

Treatment with Chinese Herbal Medicine

Citations that included interventions using CHM were identified and categorised into those that were related to 'possible post-stroke spasticity', since they were used to treat one of the search terms and there were no reasons to exclude them as unlikely to have been associated with post-stroke motor function impairment. A subset of these citations, which mentioned specific symptoms similar to spasticity, was considered to be 'more likely' to have referred to post-stroke spasticity. The most frequently used formulas and herbs are summarised below under these two levels.

Most Frequent Formulas in 'Possibly Post-stroke Spasticity' Citations

Among the 1,028 CHM citations included in this pool, 117 treatments were combinations of multiple herbs without formula names. A total of 472 named formulae were identified, with 162 of them being described in multiple citations. The most frequently seen formulas are listed in Table 3.4. Since the ingredients of one formula may change over time or be modified from different books, the ingredients from the earliest citation are presented in Table 3.4.

All the formulae were orally ingested. The most frequently used CHM formulas among these citations are *Da qin jiao tang* 大秦艽汤, followed by modified *Si wu tang* 四物汤加减, *Xiao xu ming tang* 小续命汤, *San huang tang* 三黄汤 (*Qian jin sang huang tang* 千金三黄汤), modified *Liu jun zi tang* 六君子汤加减, *Xu ming tang* 续命汤 and *Di huang yin zi* 地黄饮子. Although *Xiao xu ming tang* 小续命汤 and *Xu ming tang* 续命汤 are named similarly, their herb ingredients are quite different; therefore they are not considered to be a formula and its modified version. None of the formulas are recommended in current key textbooks and clinical practice guidelines (see Chapter 2). This may be because firstly, the understanding of the aetiology of stroke has changed over time. As mentioned before, stroke was initially defined as external Wind attack, and later Kidney

Table 3.4 Most Frequent Formulas in 'Possible Post-stroke Spasticity' Citations

Formula Name	Herb Ingredients	Number of Citations (*n*)
Da qin jiao tang 大秦艽汤	*Qin jiao* 秦艽, *gan cao* 甘草, *chuan xiong* 川芎, *dang gui* 当归, *bai shao* 白芍, *xi xin* 细辛, *qiang huo* 羌活, *fang feng* 防风, *huang qin* 黄芩, *shi gao* 石膏, *bai zhi* 白芷, *bai zhu* 白术, *shu di huang* 熟地黄, *fu ling* 茯苓 and *du huo* 独活 (*Wei Sheng Bao Jian* 卫生宝鉴 c. 1281).	25
Modified *Si wu tang* 四物汤加减	*Dang gui* 当归, *chuan xiong* 川芎, *bai shao* 白芍, *shu di huang* 熟地黄, *tao ren* 桃仁, *hong hua* 红花, *zhu li* 竹沥 and *sheng jiang* 生姜 (*Ren Shu Bian Lan* 仁术便览 c. 1585).	22
Xiao xu ming tang 小续命汤	*Ma huang* 麻黄, *rou gui* 肉桂, *gan cao* 甘草, *ren shen* 人参, *bai shao* 白芍, *chuan xiong* 川芎, *huang qin* 黄芩, *fang feng* 防风, *dang dui* 当归, *shi gao* 石膏, *bai zhu* 白术, *sheng jiang* 生姜, *fu zi* 附子, *xing ren* 杏仁, *hai zao* 海藻 and pork (*Wai Tai Mi Yao* 外台秘要 c. 752).	17
San huang tang 三黄汤 (*Qian jin sang huang tang* 千金三黄汤)	*Ma huang* 麻黄, *huang qi* 黄芪, *huang qin* 黄芩, *du huo* 独活, *xi xin* 细辛 (*Bei Ji Qian Jin Yao Fang* 备急千金要方 c. 652).	13
Modified *Liu jun zi tang* 六君子汤加减	*Ren shen* 人参, *bai zhu* 白术, *fu ling* 茯苓, *gan cao* 甘草, *chen pi* 陈皮 and *ban xia* 半夏 (*Chi Shui Xuan Zhu* 赤水玄珠 c. 1584).	11
Xu ming tang 续命汤	*Ma huang* 麻黄, *gui zhi* 桂枝, *ren shen* 人参, *dang gui* 当归, *chuan xiong* 川芎, *shi gao* 石膏, *xing ren* 杏仁, *sheng jiang* 生姜 and *gan cao* 甘草 (*Gu Jin Yi Tong Da Quan* 古今医统大全 c. 1556).	10
Di huang yin zi 地黄饮子	*Sheng di huang* 生地黄, *shu di huang* 熟地黄, *shi chang pu* 石菖蒲, *ba ji tian* 巴戟天, *fu zi* 附子, *rou gui* 肉桂, *shi hu* 石斛, *fu ling* 茯苓, *yuan zhi* 远志, *mai men dong* 麦门冬, *wu wei zi* 五味子, *bo he* 薄荷 and *shan zhu yu* 山茱萸 (*Zheng Zhi Zhun Sheng* 证治准绳 c. 1602).	9

(*Continued*)

Table 3.4 (*Continued*)

Formula Name	Herb Ingredients	Number of Citations (*n*)
Wu yao shun qi san 乌药顺气散	*Wu yao* 乌药, *chen pi* 陈皮, *ma huang* 麻黄, *jiang can* 僵蚕, *chuan xiong* 川芎, *zhi shi* 枳实, *gan cao* 甘草, *jie geng* 桔梗, *bai zhi* 白芷, *sheng jiang* 生姜 and *da zao* 大枣 (*Qi Xiao Liang Fang* 奇效良方 c. 1470).	8
Tian ma wan 天麻丸	1. *Tian ma* 天麻, *di yu* 地榆, *mo yao* 没药, *xuan shen* 玄参, *fu zi* 附子, *she xiang* 麝香, *feng mi* 蜂蜜 and *jiu* 酒; 2. *Tian ma* 天麻, *xuan shen* 玄参, *fang feng* 防风, *di yu* 地榆, *bo he* 薄荷, *fu zi* 附子, *niu xi* 牛膝, *zao jiao* 皂荚, *niu huang* 牛黄, *long nao* 龙脑, *jiu* 酒, *feng mi* 蜂蜜 and *fu ping* 浮萍 (*Sheng Ji Zong Lu* 圣济总录 c. 1117).	8

(1) Formula ingredients are based on the earliest book within the group of included citations; (2) Formulas with the same name can vary in their ingredients, and the same combination of ingredients may have different names. In this data, formulas with the same name that have variations in a few ingredients are grouped together, while those with large variations in ingredients are separated. Also, formulas with the same ingredients but different names have been grouped together; (3) The use of some herbs/ingredients may be restricted in some countries, e.g. herbs such as *fu zi* 附子, *wu tou* 乌头 and *xi xin* 细辛 can be toxic, and some may be restricted under the Convention on International Trade in Endangered Species of Wild Fauna and Flora (CITES) e.g. *she xiang* 麝香. Readers are advised to comply with relevant regulations.

deficiency and Phlegm also played an important role in the aetiology. Secondly, citations which were considered to be treating stroke with motor and function impairment in general were included in this level of analysis, thus these formulas may not be particularly focused on post-stroke spasticity. However, although these formulas are not consistent with those recommended in key textbooks and clinical practice guidelines (see Chapter 2), they may have some similarity in terms of the key herbs. Therefore, examining the actual herb ingredients is more meaningful.

Most Frequent Herbs in 'Possibly Post-stroke Spasticity' Citations

The herb frequency analysis showed that there were a total of 473 different ingredients used in the citations included in this pool. The top 20 most frequently used herbs are listed in Table 3.5. It is noted that *jiu* 酒 was one of the most frequently used ingredients which was used in preparations to process the herbs. Also, *jiu* 酒 has the function of warming and smoothing meridians, which could be beneficial for treating post-stroke motor and functional impairment.

Being used in 429 included citations, the most common herb was *dang gui* 当归. *Dang gui* 当归 is commonly used as a Blood nourishing and moving herb to remove Blood stasis. The second most frequent herb was *fang feng* 防风. Since it was believed that stroke was caused by a sudden Wind attack, the use of *fang feng* 防风 was for the purpose of eliminating Wind. The third frequently used herb was *gan cao* 甘草; this is not surprising because *gan cao* 甘草 is frequently used to harmonise all ingredients in a formula.

Among the 20 most frequently used herbs, some have the function of nourishing Blood and removing Blood stasis, e.g. *dang gui* 当归, *chuan xiong* 川芎 and *di huang* 地黄; some herbs could tonify *qi*, Spleen or Kidney, e.g. *fu zi* 附子, *wu tou* 乌头, *rou gui* 肉桂, *ren shen* 人参, *bai zhu* 白术, *fu ling* 茯苓 and ginger 生姜; some herbs may eliminate Wind, e.g. *fang feng* 防风, *qiang huo* 羌活, *ma huang* 麻黄 and *xi xin* 细辛; and some herbs could work in unblocking meridians, e.g. *tian ma* 天麻 and *niu xi* 牛膝.

Fu zi 附子, *wu tou* 乌头 and *xi xin* 细辛 are shown in the top 20 most frequently used herbs. It is believed that the use of *fu zi* 附子 and *wu tou* 乌头 was for the purpose of warming and assisting the removal of dampness/Phlegm. While *xi xin* 细辛 is often used in formulas eliminating external Wind, this reflects the fact that external Wind was considered as the causality of stroke in Chinese history. It should be noted that these herbs are currently restricted in some countries due to their toxicity. In fact, some methods of detoxing *fu*

Table 3.5 Most Frequent Herbs in 'Possible Post-stroke Spasticity' Citations

Herb Name	Scientific Name	No. of Citations (*n*)
Dang gui 当归	*Angelica sinensis* (Oliv.) Diels	429
Fang feng 防风	*Saposhnikovia divaricata* (Turcz.) Schischk.	414
Gan cao 甘草	*Glycyrrhizae* Radix et Rhizoma	396
Sheng jiang, jiang 生姜, 姜	*Zingiber officinale* (Willd.) Rosc. (fresh or dried rhizome)	376
Chuan xiong 川芎	*Ligusticum chuanxiong* Hort.	368
Fu zi 附子	*Aconitum carmichaeli* Debx.	333
Rou gui 肉桂, 肉桂枝, 官桂	*Cinnamomum cassia* Presl	293
Ren shen 人参	*Panax ginsng* C.A. Mey.	288
Ma huang 麻黄	*Ephedra spp.*	271
Di huang (*shu di huang/ sheng di huang/dihuang*) 地黄 (熟地黄/生地黄/地黄)	*Rehmannia glutinosa* Libosch.	258 (172/73/13)
Bai zhu 白术	*Atractylodes macrocephala* Koidz.	251
Qiang huo 羌活	*Notopterygium incisum Ting ex H. T. Chang*	237
Fu ling 茯苓	*Poria cocos* (Schw.) Wolf	222
Jiu 酒	Alcohol	215
Du huo 独活	*Angelica pubescens* Maxim. f. *biserrata* Shan et Yuan	215
Bai shao 白芍	*Paeonia lactiflora* Pall.	210
Tian ma 天麻	*Gastrodia elata* Bl.	204
Wu tou/chuan wu/cao wu 乌头, 川乌, 草乌	1. *Aconitum carmichaeli* Debx. 2. *Aconitum kusnezoffii* Reichb.	167
Xi xin 细辛	1. *Asarum heterotropoides* Fr. Schmidt var. *mandshuricum* (Maxim) Kitag. 2. *Asarum sieboldii* Miq. var. *seoulense* Nakai 3. *Asarum sieboldii* Miq.	151
Niu xi 牛膝	*Cyathula officinalis* Kuan	150

The use of some herbs such as *fu zi* 附子, *wu tou* 乌头 and *xi xin* 细辛 may be restricted in some countries. Readers are advised to comply with relevant regulations.

zi 附子 and *wu tou* 乌头 had been introduced in ancient China while the toxicity of *xi xin* 细辛 was not mentioned. It was recorded in the book *Dan Xi Xin Fa* 丹溪心法 written in 1347 AD that, boiling *fu zi* 附子 and *wu tou* 乌头 with urine could reduce their toxicity (凡用乌、附, 必用童便煮过, 以杀其毒).

Most Frequent Formulas in 'Likely Post-stroke Spasticity' Citations

The 'likely post-stroke spasticity citations' were defined as those treating post-stroke motor and functional impairment with a particular focus on spasticity symptoms. In total, 232 citations were judged applicable in this category based on our analysis of symptoms' description. They were obtained from a total of 76 books, with the most common ones being *Pu Ji Fang* 普济方 (c. 1406) (*n* = 34), *Tai Ping Sheng Hui Fang* 太平圣惠方 (c. 992) (*n* = 27), *Sheng Ji Zong Lu* 圣济总录 (c. 1117) (*n* = 16), *Ji Yang Gang Mu* 济阳纲目 (c. 1626) (*n* = 9), *Tai Ping Hui Min He Ji Ju Fang* 太平惠民和剂局方 (c. 1151) (*n* = 8), *Ru Men Shi Qin* 儒门事亲 (c. 1228) (*n* = 7), *Yi Xue Gang Mu* 医学纲目 (c. 1565) (*n* = 7), *Bei Ji Qian Jin Yao Fang* 备急千金要方 (c. 652) (*n* = 7), *Qi Xiao Liang Fang* 奇效良方 (c. 1470) (*n* = 7) and *Wai Tai Mi Yao* 外台秘要 (c. 752) (*n* = 5).

A total of 151 formulas were found from the 232 citations, with 30 formulas appearing on more than one occasion. The most frequent formulas being introduced in multiple citations are *San huang tang* 三黄汤 (*Qian jin san huang tang* 千金三黄汤) (*n* = 7), *Xu ming tang* 续命汤 (*n* = 7), *Xiao xu ming tang* 小续命汤 (*n* = 6), *Xing feng tang* 省风汤 (*n* = 5), *Fang feng san* 防风散 (*n* = 4), *Da jin ya jiu* 大金牙酒 (*n* = 3), *Zuo jing wan* 左经丸 (*n* = 3), *Du huo san* 独活散 (*n* = 3) and *Qin jiao sheng ma tang* 秦艽升麻汤 (*n* = 3) (see Table 3.6). Except for *San huang tang* 三黄汤 (*Qian jin san huang tang* 千金三黄汤), *Xu ming tang* 续命汤 and *Xiao xu ming tang* 小续命汤, the other formulas are not shown in the 'possible' pool (Table 3.4). However, due to the small number of citations identified, the function of these formulas could not be confirmed.

Table 3.6 Most Frequent Formulas in 'Likely Post-stroke Spasticity' Citations

Formula Name	Herb Ingredients	Number of Citations (*n*)
San huang tang 三黄汤 (*Qian jin sang huang tang* 千金三黄汤)	*Ma huang* 麻黄, *huang qi* 黄芪, *huang qin* 黄芩, *du huo* 独活 and *xi xin* 细辛 (*Bei Ji Qian Jin Yao Fang* 备急千金要方 c. 652).	12
Xu ming tang 续命汤	*Ma huang* 麻黄, *gui zhi* 桂枝, *ren shen* 人参, *dang gui* 当归, *chuan xiong* 川芎, *shi gao* 石膏, *xing ren* 杏仁, *sheng jiang* 生姜 and *gan cao* 甘草 (*Gu Jin Yi Tong Da Quan* 古今医统大全 c. 1556).	7
Xiao xu ming tang 小续命汤	*Ma huang* 麻黄, *rou gui* 肉桂, *gan cao* 甘草, *ren shen* 人参, *bai shao* 白芍, *chuan xiong* 川芎, *huang qin* 黄芩, *fang feng* 防风, *dang dui* 当归, *shi gao* 石膏, *bai zhu* 白术, *sheng jiang* 生姜, *fu zi* 附子, *xing ren* 杏仁, *hai zao* 海藻 and pork (*Wai Tai Mi Yao* 外台秘要 c. 752).	6
Xing feng tang 省风汤	*Fang feng* 防风, *tian nan xing* 天南星, *ban xia* 半夏, *huang qin* 黄芩 and *gan cao* 甘草 (*Tai Ping Hui Min He Ji Ju Fang* 太平惠民和剂局方 c. 1078).	5
Fang feng san 防风散	*Fang feng* 防风, *bai zhu* 白术, *chuan xiong* 川芎, *xi xin* 细辛, *qiang huo* 羌活, *yin yu* 茵芋, *niu xi* 牛膝, *gou ji* 狗脊, *bei xie* 萆薢, *yi yi ren* 薏苡仁, *ma huang* 麻黄, *xing ren* 杏仁, *tian ma* 天麻, *rou gui* 肉桂, *sheng jiang* 生姜 and *fu zi* 附子 (*Tai Ping Sheng Hui Fang* 太平圣惠方 c. 992).	4
Da jin ya jiu 大金牙酒	*Fu zi* 附子, *tian xiong* 天雄, *ren shen* 人参, *rou cong rong* 肉苁蓉, *fu ling* 茯苓, *dang gui* 当归, *fang feng* 防风, *huang qi* 黄芪, *shan yao* 山药, *xi xin* 细辛 and *rou gui* 肉桂 (*Bei Ji Qian Jin Yao Fang* 备急千金要方 c. 652).	3
Zuo jing wan 左经丸	*Wu tou* 乌头, *gei dou* 黑豆, *ban mao* 斑蝥 and *jiu* 酒 (*Pu Ji Fang* 普济方 c. 1390).	3

(*Continued*)

Table 3.6 (*Continued*)

Formula Name	Herb Ingredients	Number of Citations (*n*)
Du huo san 独活散	*Du huo* 独活, *zhi shi* 枳实, *chuan xiong* 川芎, *fang feng* 防风, *dang gui* 当归, *xi xin* 细辛, *rou gui* 肉桂, *tian ma* 天麻 and *zhu li* 竹沥 (*Tai Ping Sheng Hui Fang* 太平圣惠方 c. 992).	3
Qin jiao sheng ma tang 秦艽升麻汤	*Sheng ma* 升麻, *tian hua fen* 天花粉, *gan cao* 甘草, *bai shao* 白芍, *ren shen* 人参, *qin jiao* 秦艽, *bai zhi* 白芷, *fang feng* 防风, *gui zhi* 桂枝 and *cong bai* 葱白 (*Yi Xue Gang Mu* 医学纲目 c. 1565).	3

(1) Formula ingredients are based on the earliest book within the group of included citations; (2) Formulas with the same name can vary in their ingredients and the same combination of ingredients may have different names. In this data, formulas with the same name that have variations in a few ingredients are grouped together, while those with large variations in ingredients are separated. Also, formulas with the same ingredients but different names have been grouped together; (3) The use of some herbs/ingredients may be restricted in some countries, e.g. herbs such as *fu zi* 附子, *wu tou* 乌头 and *xi xin* 细辛 can be toxic, and some may be restricted under the Convention on International Trade in Endangered Species of Wild Fauna and Flora (CITES). Readers are advised to comply with relevant regulations.

Most Frequent Herbs in 'Likely Post-stroke Spasticity' Citations

By analysing the ingredients of the 232 citations, a total of 298 herbs were found. The most frequently used 20 herbs are presented in Table 3.7.

These herbs are consistent with the 20 most frequently used herbs of the 'possible post-stroke spasticity' citations, except for *quan xie* 全蝎 (see Table 3.5). *Quan xie* 全蝎 is said to have the function of relieving spasm and pain. However, it should be used in small dosages since it contains buthotoxin.

Representative Case Report

Our search identified six case reports using CHM to manage post-stroke motor and functional impairment with spasticity. Different CHM formulas were used in these case reports. One citation from a book of the Ming dynasty (*Shou Shi Bao Yuan* 寿世保元, c. 1615)

Table 3.7 Most Frequent Herbs in 'Likely Post-stroke Spasticity' Citations

Herb Name	Scientific Name	No. of Citations (n)
Fang feng 防风	*Saposhnikovia divaricata* (Turcz.) Schischk.	115
Dang gui 当归	*Angelica sinensis* (Oliv.) Diels	96
Chuan xiong 川芎	*Ligusticum chuanxiong* Hort.	94
Fu zi 附子	*Aconitum carmichaeli* Debx.	86
Gan cao 甘草	*Glycyrrhizae* Radix et Rhizoma	86
Ma huang 麻黄	Ephedrae Herba	78
Rou gui 肉桂 (肉桂枝, 官桂)	*Cinnamomum cassia* Presl	72
Jiang 姜 (生姜)	*Zingiber officinale* (Willd.) Rosc. (fresh or dried rhizome)	68
Du huo 独活	*Angelica pubescens* Maxim. f. *biserrata* Shan et Yuan	65
Ren shen 人参	*Panax ginsng* C.A. Mey.	64
Qiang huo 羌活	*Notopterygium incisum Ting ex H. T. Chang*	*52*
Jiu 酒	Alcohol	51
Bai zhu 白术	*Atractylodes macrocephala* Koidz.	50
Huang qin 黄芩	*Scutellaria baicalensis* Georgi	49
Niu xi 牛膝	*Cyathula officinalis* Kuan	46
Wu tou 乌头 (川乌, 草乌)	1. *Aconitum carmichaeli* Debx. 2. *Aconitum kusnezoffii* Reichb.	44
Tian ma 天麻	*Gastrodia elata* Bl.	42
Bai shao 白芍	*Paeonia lactiflora* Pall.	39
Xi xin 细辛	1. *Asarum heterotropoides* Fr. Schmidt var. *mandshuricum* (Maxim) Kitag. 2. *Asarum sieboldii* Miq. var. *seoulense* Nakai 3. *Asarum sieboldii* Miq.	39
Quan xie 全蝎	*Buthus martensii* Karsch	36

The use of some herbs such as *fu zi* 附子, *wu tou* 乌头 and *xi xin* 细辛 may be restricted in some countries. Readers are advised to comply with relevant regulations.

reported that a CHM formula (*Shi guo gong jin jiu liang fang* 史国公浸酒良方) cured a patient who had suffered from post-stroke hemiplegia and spasticity for more than ten years. Considering this formula had not been cited by other books, the effectiveness could not be further confirmed.

Discussion of Chinese Herbal Medicine for Post-stroke Spasticity

For the treatment of post-stroke motor and functional impairment possibly including spasticity, a total of 1,028 citations were identified. Of these, 232 citations addressed spasticity symptoms and therefore were selected as the most representative pool.

Among the citations 'possibly referring to post-stroke spasticity', a total of 472 named CHM formulas, containing 473 different ingredients, were identified, with 162 formulas being introduced by multiple citations. Focusing on the symptoms of spasticity, a total of 151 named formulas were found from 232 citations. The most frequently used ones were *San huang tang* 三黄汤, *Xu ming tang* 续命汤, *Xiao xu ming tang* 小续命汤, *Qian jin san huang tang* 千金三黄汤, *Xing feng tang* 省风汤, *Fang feng san* 防风散, *Da jin ya jiu* 大金牙酒, *Zuo jing wan* 左经丸, *Du huo san* 独活散 and *Qin jiao sheng ma tang* 秦艽升麻汤. These formulas are not consistent with those recommended by current clinical guidelines or textbooks (see Chapter 2). This could be explained by the fact that the understanding of stroke's aetiology in CM has changed over time. On the other hand, although these formulas are not recommended in contemporary literature for treating post-stroke spasticity, the most frequently used herbs showed the main functions of nourishing Blood and removing Blood stasis, tonifying *qi* 气, Spleen or Kidney, eliminating Wind and unblocking meridians. These functions are similar to the treatment principles used in current practice. In particular, the treatment purposes of tonifying *qi* 气, removing Blood stasis and opening up meridians are consistent with that of *Bu yang huan wu tang* 补阳还五汤, the key formula being recommended by clinical guidelines to treat post-stroke motor and functional impairment.

It has been noted that some herbs frequently used in history are no longer in use in current clinical practice. For example, *she xiang* 麝香 is produced from an internationally endangered animal and is restricted under the provisions of CITES. In addition, some herbs such as *fu zi* 附子, *wu tou* 乌头 and *xi xin* 细辛 may be restricted in some countries due to their toxicity. In fact, the toxicity of *fu zi* 附子 and *wu tou* 乌头 had been noted in classical literature. The book *Dan Xi Xin Fa* 丹溪心法, written in 1347 AD, introduced a method for reducing their toxicity — by being boiled in urine (凡用乌、附, 必用童便煮过, 以杀其毒), although the mechanism of urine for detoxification has not been proven.

Acupuncture and Related Therapies

A total of 162 citations stated acupuncture or moxibustion treatments for symptoms 'possibly related to post-stroke spasticity'. They were found in 46 books;, the most cited ones are *Pu Ji Fang – Zhen Jiu* 普济方•针灸 (c. 1406) ($n = 20$), *Gu Jin Yi Tong Da Quan* 古今医统大全 (c. 1556) ($n = 15$), *Mian Xue Tang Zhen Jiu Ji Cheng* 勉学堂针灸集成 (c. 1874) ($n = 15$), *Lei Jing Tu Yi* 类经图翼 (c. 1624) ($n = 10$), *Zhen Jiu Da Cheng* 针灸大成 (c. 1601) ($n = 10$), *Tai Ping Sheng Hui Fang* 太平圣惠方 (c. 992) ($n = 9$), *Zhen Jiu Ju Ying* 针灸聚英 (c. 1529) ($n = 8$), *Sheng Ji Zong Lu* 圣济总录 (c. 1117) ($n = 7$) and *Zhen Fang Liu Ji* 针方六集 (c. 1618) ($n = 6$).

Frequency of Treatment Citations by Dynasty

Similar to the CHM citations, the majority of these citations were identified in books from the Ming dynasty (c. 1369–1644) and Qing dynasty (c. 1645–1911). The earliest treatment citations were from *Huang Di Ming Tang Jiu Jing* 黄帝明堂灸经 (Tang dynasty), and the most recent citations were from the book *Jin Zhen Mi Zhuan* 金针秘传 (published in 1937). Five citations were from books without known publishing years, and one citation was from a Japanese acupuncture textbook published in the Qing dynasty (Table 3.8).

Table 3.8 Dynastic Distribution of Treatment Citations

Dynasty	No. of Treatment Citations
Before Tang dynasty (before 618)	0
Tang and 5 dynasties (618–960)	6
Song and Jin dynasties (961–1271)	25
Yuan dynasty (1272–1368)	8
Ming dynasty (1369–1644)	79
Qing dynasty (1645–1911)	36
Min Guo/Republic of China (1912–1949)	2
Others	5 unknowns, 1 Japan*
Total	**162**

*Chinese medicine books published in Japan.

Treatment with Acupuncture-related Therapies

Of these 162 acupuncture citations, 111 citations stated that a particular acupuncture point could be used for treating certain clinical conditions or symptoms. There were two citations that recorded clinical case reports.

Frequency of Acupuncture Points in 'Possibly Post-stroke Spasticity' Acupuncture Citations

A total of 96 acupuncture points were found in the citations. The top 20 are presented in Table 3.9.

These acupuncture points can be grouped according to their locations and functions as below:

- Upper limb: LI11 *Quchi* 曲池, LI15 *Jianyu* 肩髃, LI10 *Shousanli* 手三里, LU7 *Lieque* 列缺, LI4 *Hegu* 合谷 and GB21 *Jianjing* 肩井;
- Lower limb: GB31 *Fengshi* 风市, GB30 *Huantiao* 环跳, B34 *Yanglingquan* 阳陵泉, BL60 *Kunlun* 昆仑, ST36 *Zusanli* 足三里, BL40 *Weizhong* 委中, GB39 *Xuanzhong* 悬钟, KI6 *Zhaohai* 照海, GB38 *Yangfu* 阳辅 and GB40 *Qiuxu* 丘墟;
- Facial area: CV24 *Chengjiang* 承浆, GB3 *Shangguan* 上关, ST4 *Dicang* 地仓, GB2 *Tinghui* 听会 and ST6 *Jiache* 颊车.

Table 3.9 Most Frequently Used Acupuncture Points in 'Possible Post-stroke Spasticity' Acupuncture Citations

Acupuncture Points	No. of Citations (*n*)
LI11 *Quchi* 曲池	41
LI15 *Jianyu* 肩髃	32
GV20 *Baihui* 百会	24
LI10 *Shousanli* 手三里	22
GB31 *Fengshi* 风市	20
GB30 *Huantiao* 环跳	19
LU7 *Lieque* 列缺	19
GB39 *Xuanzhong* 悬钟	18
LI4 *Hegu* 合谷	15
GB34 *Yanglingquan* 阳陵泉	15
BL60 *Kunlun* 昆仑	12
CV24 *Chengjiang* 承浆	11
ST36 *Zusanli* 足三里	11
GB21 *Jianjing* 肩井	10
BL40 *Weizhong* 委中	7
GB3 *Shangguan* 上关	7
ST4 *Dicang* 地仓	6
KI6 *Zhaohai* 照海	6
GV16 *Fengfu* 风府	5
GB40 *Qiuxu* 丘墟	5
ST6 *Jiache* 颊车	5
BL15 *Xinshu* 心俞	5
GB2 *Tinghui* 听会	5
GB20 *Fengchi* 风池	5
GB38 *Yangfu* 阳辅	5

Other points reflect treatment principles based on their functions:

- To clear mind and *Shen* 神: GV20 *Baihui* 百会, and BL15 *Xinshu* 心俞;
- To eliminate wind: GV16 *Fengfu* 风府 and GB20 *Fengchi* 风池.

However, these citations are not specifically for post-stroke spasticity; hence these points could be used in general acupuncture treatment for post-stroke hemiplegia.

Most of the included citations (n = 111) were extracted from acupuncture books. In the ancient acupuncture books, acupuncture points were introduced under each meridian section, with the information of locations, disease to be treated, depth of needling and time, duration or dosage of moxibustion etc., being provided. For example, 'GB30 *Huantiao* 环跳 is located at…, 50 moxibustion, or needling of one *cun* 寸, needle could be kept for 10 breath's time, this point can be used to treat conditions such as …' (*Pu ji fang-Zhen jiu* 普济方•针灸, c. 1406).

One citation, from a book published in the Qing dynasty, reported a clinical case of using CHM and acupuncture to treat an acute stroke. The details are as follows: 'a 68-year-old woman, symptoms presented are stiffness and muscular contracture of left side limbs, stiffness of tongue, aphasia, and dysphagia. This is caused by stroke and Phlegm. After taking CHM for 20 doses, the muscular contracture of left side limbs and aphasia remained. In this case, acupuncture is needed. Needling EX-UE3 *Zhongquan* 中泉 and SJ6 *Zhigou* 支沟 could reduce the Phlegm, the patient then keep taking CHM for another 70 doses until all symptoms were resolved' (*Wu Ju Tong Yi An* 吴鞠通医案•中风). This case report detailed how to combine CHM and acupuncture for the management of acute stroke involving spasticity. Practitioners may consider such a method in current clinical practice.

Frequency of Acupuncture Points in 'Likely Post-stroke Spasticity' Citations

By placing the criterion of 'spasticity-specific symptoms', the pool of acupuncture citations was narrowed down to a total of 30 citations. They were obtained from 13 books: *Pu Ji Fang – Zhen Jiu* 普济方•针灸 (c. 1406) (n = 10), *Zhen jiu da cheng* 针灸大成 (c. 1601) (n = 5), *Sheng ji zong lu* 圣济总录 (c. 1117) (n = 2), *Bian Que Shen Ying Zhen Jiu Yu Long Jing* 扁鹊神应针灸玉龙经 (c. 1368) (n = 2), *Pu ji ben shi fang* 普济本事方 (c. 1132) (*n* = 2), *Zhen jiu wen da* 针灸问答 (c. 1930) (*n* = 2), *Wai tai mi yao* 外台秘要 (c. 752) (*n* = 1), *Tai ping sheng hui fang* 太平圣惠方 (c. 992) (*n* = 1), *Wu ju tong yi an* 吴鞠通医案 (c. 1798) (*n* = 1), *Jiu fang mi zhuan* 灸法秘传 (c. 1883) (*n* = 1), *Bing ji sha zhuan* 病机沙篆 (c. 1667) (*n* = 1), *Xi fang zi ming tang jiu jing* 西方子明堂灸经 (c. 1368) (*n* = 1) and *Zhen fang liu ji* 针方六集 (c. 1618) (*n* = 1). A total of 36 acupuncture points were found from these citations, with 16 points being shown in multiple citations (Table 3.10).

Of these, 13 points are consistent with the most frequently cited acupuncture points of 'possible post-stroke spasticity' citations (see Table 3.9). Three points (LI9 *Shanglian* 上廉, PC6 *Neiguan* 内关 and SI4 *Wangu* 腕骨) were not shown in Table 3.9. However, due to their very small frequency, it could not be confirmed whether these three

Table 3.10 Most Frequently Used Acupuncture Points in 'Likely Post-stroke Spasticity' Citations

Acupuncture Points	No. of Citations (*n*)
LI15 *Jianyu* 肩髃	11
LI11 *Quchi* 曲池	7
LI4 *Hegu* 合谷	5
GB30 *Huantiao* 环跳	5
LI10 *Shousanli* 手三里	4
GV20 *Baihui* 百会	4
BL60 *Kunlun* 昆仑	4
GB31 *Fengshi* 风市	3
GB34 *Yanglingquan* 阳陵泉	3
BL40 *Weizhong* 委中	3
GB21 *Jianjing* 肩井	2
LI9 *Shanglian* 上廉	2
ST36 *Zusanli* 足三里	2
LU7 *Lieque* 列缺	2
PC6 *Neiguan* 内关	2
SI4 *Wangu* 腕骨	2

points may have special treatment effects for spasticity. It seems that all these points are the common acupuncture points used for post-stroke hemiplegia.

Discussion of Acupuncture and Related Therapies for Post-stroke Spasticity

Our search of ZHYD found that acupuncture treatment for *zhong feng* 中风 dates back to the Tang dynasty and had been continually used until current clinical practice. It is found by our review that the earliest description of 'likely' post-stroke spasticity treated with acupuncture is from the book published in the Tang dynasty, *Wai Tai Mi Yao* 外台秘要 (c. 752). There was a total of 162 citations identified as acupuncture treatment for post-stroke motor and functional impairment, possibly including the symptom of spasticity. When the criteria were limited to 'spasticity-specific symptoms', 30 citations were included in the most representative pool.

A total of 96 acupuncture points were identified from all included citations. Similar to current clinical practice, the principle of selecting acupuncture points in the treatments for post-stroke motor and functional impairment is mainly choosing the points in the affected area, assisted by CM syndrome differentiation. Furthermore, 16 acupuncture points were found from the 30 citations which specifically mentioned spasticity-like symptoms. These points are commonly used ones in acupuncture treatment for post-stroke hemiplegia. Our analysis of these citations did not locate any special acupuncture point carrying anti-spasticity function.

Classical Literature in Perspective

In the history of CM, *zhong feng* 中风 was characterised as a group of symptoms of stroke. A number of terms were used referring to different stages or symptoms of stroke. Terms such as *pu ji* 仆击, *da jue* 大厥 and *po jue* 薄厥 indicated the acute stage stroke with unconsciousness; *ban shen bu sui* 半身不遂, *pian ku* 偏枯, *pian feng* 偏风 and *feng fei* 风痱 were the names of hemiplegia; aphasia was described using *yin fei* 喑痱, etc. However, there has not been a specific disease name referring to post-stroke spasticity. Spasticity was only recorded as one of the post-stroke symptoms using different terms such as *shou zu ju luan* 手足拘挛, *ju ji* 拘急, *jin luan* 筋挛, *luan suo* 挛缩, *luan bi* 挛躄, *jin mai luan ji* 筋脉挛急, *jin ji* 筋急, *chi cong* 瘛疭, *ju luan qu shen bu de* 拘挛屈伸不得 and *jiu feng ku zhi* 久风枯挚. Therefore, we screened all citations related to stroke motor and functional impairment and selected those that contained description of spasticity-like symptoms.

Zhong feng 中风, refers to 'a sudden Wind attack'. The concept of 'Wind' in stroke was initially an external pathogen which then developed to become internal Wind of Liver *yang* 阳 uprising. It was recorded in *Huang Di Nei Jing* 黄帝内经 that the causality of this disease was said to be external pathogen invasion together with *qi* 气 deficiency. Overweight/obesity was noted as a potential risk factor of *pian ku* 偏枯 in *Huang Di Nei Jing* 黄帝内经. The classification of *zhong jing* 中经, *zhong luo* 中络, *zhong zang* 中脏 and *zhong fu* 中腑 was brought out in the Han dynasty by a famous physician Zhang Zhong-Jing 张仲景 according to the severity of *zhong feng* 中风. In the Song dynasty, the causality of *zhong feng* 中风 started to be switched to internal factors. For instance, the deficiency of *zang-fu* 脏腑, *qi* 气 and Blood was emphasised to be the fundamental factor of Wind attack. In the Jin and Yuan dynasty, it was believed that *zhong feng* 中风 was caused by internal factors rather than external pathogens. Zhu Dan-Xi 朱丹溪 pointed out that *zhong feng* 中风 was the result of a combination of multiple internal pathogens including *qi* 气 and Blood deficiency, Phlegm, Blood stasis and Heat. This is consistent with the current CM theory. However, Zhu Dan-Xi 朱丹溪 claimed that the hemiplegia which happens on the different sides of the body is caused by different reasons, which is an incorrect theory due to limited knowledge in human anatomy. In the Ming dynasty, Liver *yang* 阳 upraising became the dominating aetiology of *zhong feng* 中风. The concept of 'internal Wind' caused by Liver *yang* 阳 uprising was introduced in the Qing dynasty. In the Minguo period, along with the spread of western medicine knowledge, Chinese physician Zhang Xi-Chun 张锡纯 adopted the two types of stroke (ischaemic, due to lack of blood supply; and haemorrhagic, due to bleeding) and put forward the name of *nao pin xue* 脑贫血 and *nao chong xue* 脑充血 (*Yi Xue Zhong Zhong Can Xi Lu* 医学衷中参西录, c. 1909). Nonetheless, in the long history of the development of the aetiology and causality of *zhong feng* 中风, post-stroke spasticity had never been specifically discussed.

With regard to CHM treatment recorded in classical literature, the formulas found in our review are different to those used in current clinical practice. This can be explained as follows: (1) In most classical books, the treatments of acute stage and sequelae stage were not clearly differentiated. Some of the formulas found by our search were often used in the acute stage of stroke in the past, but in current practice, CHM does not play an important role in this stage; (2) Formula names changed over time along with modification. For example, modified *Si wu tang* 四物汤加减 was a frequently used formula stated in classical literature. Being the most commonly used formula currently for post-stroke motor and functional impairment, *Bu yang huan wu tang* 补阳还五汤 is also a modified version of *Si wu tang* 四物汤 (see Chapter 2); however, it was named in the Qing dynasty. Therefore, it was identified by our search, but with very low frequency.

On the other hand, the frequently used herb ingredients are similar to what are in use currently. The function of those herbs included nourishing Blood and removing Blood stasis; tonifying *qi* 气, Spleen or Kidney; reducing Phlegm; eliminating Wind and opening up meridians. Although some toxic herbs such as *wu tou* 乌头 and *fu zi* 附子 were frequently used, some effort had been made to detoxify them. One herb, *quan xie* 全蝎, was found frequently used for spasticity-like symptoms due to its function of relieving spasm and pain.

Acupuncture and moxibustion had been used in ancient China for the treatment of post-stroke functional impairment. Our search of ZHYD found that LI15 *Jianyu* 肩髃, LI11 *Quchi* 曲池, LI4 *Hegu* 合谷 and GB30 *Huantiao* 环跳 are the most common acupuncture points used for 'likely' post-stroke spasticity. These points are still commonly used in acupuncture treatment for post-stroke hemiplegia. It seems that there was no singular point considered to have specific effects for spasticity.

Our review of classical literature did not identify *tuina* 推拿 therapy or other CM therapies as the treatment for post-stroke spasticity. Clinicians should carefully take account of the differences between the historical use and contemporary guidelines of CM. The findings provided in this chapter may be considered to assist clinical practice, but not to completely guide clinical practice.

References

1. Ma KW. (2000) Acupuncture: Its place in the history of Chinese medicine. *Acupunct Med* **18(2):** 88–99.
2. White A, Ernst E. (2004) A brief history of acupuncture. *Rheumatology (Oxford)* **43(5):** 662–663.
3. May BH, Lu Y, Lu C, *et al.* (2013) Systematic assessment of the representativeness of published collections of the traditional literature on Chinese medicine. *J Altern Complement Med* **19(5)**: 403–409.
4. May BH, Lu C, Xue CC. (2012) Collections of traditional Chinese medical literature as resources for systematic searches. *J Altern Complement Med* **18(12):** 1101–1107.
5. Jia Hong Science and Technology Development Co. Ltd. (2014) *Zhong Hua Yi Dian* 中华医典 (ZHYD) [*Encyclopaedia of Traditional Chinese Medicine,* 5th ed.] Hunan Electronic and Audio-Visual Publishing House, Changsha.
6. 吴朋騑. (2005) 黄芪桂枝五物汤治疗中风的现代文献研究 (Thesis). 北京中医药大学.
7. 周仲英. (2007) 中医内科学. 中国中医药出版社.
8. 张伯礼. (2012) 中医内科学. 人民卫生出版社.
9. 田德禄, 蔡淦. (2013) 中医内科学. 上海科学技术出版社.
10. 王永炎, 谢雁鸣. (2010) 实用中风病康复学. 人民卫生出版社.
11. 中国中医科学院. (2011) 中医循证临床实践指南:中医内科分册. 中国中医药出版社.
12. 高驰, 朱建平. (2014) '中风' 病名源流考. 中华中医药杂志 **(05):** 1298–1303.
13. 郜峦, 王键. (2009) 中风病病因病机的源流及发展. 中国中医急症 **(08):** 1279–1281.

14. 龚彪, 邹敏, 罗华丽. (2006) 从中风的诊断探讨中医的病名诊断. 陕西中医学院学报 **(02):** 11–12.
15. 黄伟贞. (2014) 西医脑出血与中医中风病病名诊断的对比研究. 现代中西医结合杂志 **(07):** 690–692.
16. 金栋. (2009) '卒中' 病名考. 世界中西医结合杂志 **(03):** 156–158.
17. 金栋. (2009) 古病名 '痱病' 探源. 世界中西医结合杂志 **(05):** 310–311.
18. 李红香. (2011) 基于中医文献的中风病研究 (Thesis). 南京中医药大学.
19. 李红香, 戴慎. (2011) 中风病名探源. 辽宁中医药大学学报 **(04):** 158–159.
20. 李长君. (2007) 针灸治疗中风病的文献研究 (Thesis). 黑龙江中医药大学.
21. 梁天坚. (2015) 叶天士痱中病名及证治简析. 江苏中医药 **(08):** 7–8.
22. 刘伍立, 欧阳建军, 黄博辉. (2006) 中医文献对中风病的阐述与述评. 针灸临床杂志 **(10):** 5–8, 66.
23. 王春虎, 张运克. (2014) 中风病名新解. 中医临床研究 **(31):** 47–48.
24. 王建华. (1997) 真中风类中风源流概述. 河北中医 **(04):** 45–47.
25. 温春胜. (2013) 中风病中西医病名诊断的对比研究 (Thesis). 广西医科大学.
26. 徐木林. (1996) 中风之古与今. 辽宁中医杂志 **(06):** 253–254.
27. 许玉皎. (2011) 中风病名分析及现代中风病诊断. 中医药导报 **(05):** 6–8.
28. 杨海涛, 张冬梅, 谢天. (2014) 中风病名溯源. 中国社区医师 **(06):** 10–11.
29. 张碧生. (2012) 中风源流考辩及其辨证论治规律 (Thesis). 山东中医药大学.
30. 赵永辰. (2008) '中风' 病名探源及病机沿革. 中华中医药杂志 **(04):** 290–292.
31. 赵正孝. (2003) 中医中风病的诊治思想及源流研究 (Thesis). 湖南中医学院.

4

Methods for Evaluating Clinical Evidence

OVERVIEW

This chapter describes the methods used to identify and evaluate a range of Chinese medicine interventions for post-stroke spasticity in clinical studies. Studies identified through a comprehensive search were assessed against eligibility criteria. A review of the methodological quality of the studies was undertaken using standardised methods. Results from included studies were evaluated to provide an estimate of the effects of a range of Chinese medicine therapies.

Introduction

The use of Chinese medicine (CM) for post-stroke spasticity has been well described in contemporary literature and in classical CM. Systematic reviews have been conducted to evaluate the efficacy and safety of CM treatment for post-stroke spasticity. This chapter presents the methodologies of examining the efficacy and safety of CM interventions (Table 4.1) for post-stroke spasticity in clinical studies. The evidence is presented for the following types of CM interventions:

- Chinese herbal medicine (CHM) (Chapter 5);
- Acupuncture and related therapies (Chapter 7);
- Other CM therapies (Chapter 8);
- Combination CM therapies e.g. CHM plus acupuncture (Chapter 9).

Table 4.1 Chinese Medicine Interventions Included in Clinical Evidence Evaluation

Category	Intervention
CHM	Oral or topical.
Acupuncture and related therapies	Acupuncture, acupressure, electroacupuncture and moxibustion.
Other Chinese medicine therapies	*Tuina* 推拿 (Chinese massage) therapy.
Chinese medicine combination therapies	Combination therapies are defined as two or more Chinese medicine interventions from different categories administered together e.g. CHM plus acupuncture, or CHM plus *tuina* 推拿 therapy.

Abbreviations: CHM – Chinese herbal medicine.

References to clinical trials were obtained and assessed by an expert group. Randomised controlled trials (RCTs), non-randomised controlled clinical trials (CCTs) and non-controlled studies were evaluated in detail, separately. Controlled clinical trials were evaluated using the same approach as RCTs. Meta-analyses were conducted for the RCTs and CCTs, but not for non-controlled studies. Evidence from non-controlled studies is more difficult to evaluate; therefore the approach was taken to describe the characteristics of the study, details of the intervention and any adverse events. References to included studies are indicated by a letter followed by a number. Studies of CHM are indicated by an 'H' e.g. H1; studies of acupuncture and related therapies indicated by an 'A' e.g. A1; studies of other CM therapies indicated by an 'O' e.g. O1; and studies of combination CM therapies (see Table 4.1) indicated by a 'C' e.g. C1.

Search Strategy

Comprehensive searches from English- and Chinese-language databases were conducted following the methods described in the Cochrane Handbook of Systematic Reviews.[1] English-language databases included PubMed, Excerpta Medica Database (Embase), Cumulative Index of Nursing and Allied Health Literature (CINAHL),

Cochrane Central Register of Controlled Trials (CENTRAL) including the Cochrane Library, and Allied and Complementary Medicine Database (AMED). Chinese-language databases included China BioMedical Literature (CBM), China National Knowledge Infrastructure (CNKI), Chonqing VIP (CQVIP) and Wanfang. Databases were searched from their inception to May 2015. No restrictions were applied. Search terms were mapped to controlled vocabulary (where applicable), in addition to being searched as keywords.

To conduct a comprehensive search of the literature, searches were run according to the study design (reviews, controlled trials and non-controlled studies). This was done for each of the three intervention types (CHM, acupuncture and related therapies, and other CM therapies) resulting in nine searches in each of the nine databases:

1. CHM — reviews;
2. CHM — controlled trials (randomised and non-randomised);
3. CHM — non-controlled studies;
4. Acupuncture and related therapies — reviews;
5. Acupuncture and related therapies — controlled trials (randomised and non-randomised);
6. Acupuncture and related therapies — non-controlled studies;
7. Other CM therapies — reviews;
8. Other CM therapies — controlled trials (randomised and non-randomised);
9. Other CM therapies — non-controlled studies.

Studies of combination CM therapies were identified through the above searches. In addition to electronic databases, reference lists of systematic reviews and included studies were searched for additional publications. Clinical trial registries were searched to identify clinical trials which were ongoing or completed, and where required, trial investigators were contacted to obtain data. The searched trial registries included the Australian New Zealand Clinical Trial Registry (ANZCTR), the Chinese Clinical Trial Registry (ChiCTR), the European Union Clinical Trials Register (EU-CTR), and the US National Institutes of Health register (ClinicalTrials.gov).

Inclusion Criteria

Studies to be included in our systematic analyses are controlled studies with, or without, randomisation and non-controlled studies (cohort, case series and case studies) that had employed a CM therapy as a test intervention and reported pre-defined outcomes which are relevant to post-stroke spasticity.

- Participants: Patients who suffered a stroke (ischaemic or haemorrhagic type) with a confirmed diagnosis (confirmed by computed tomography or magnetic resonance imaging scan), with the development of clinical symptoms of post-stroke spasticity defined by clinical guideline;[2,3]
- Interventions: Chinese herbal medicine, acupuncture and related therapies, or other CM therapies, alone or in combination with other CM therapies or with pharmacotherapy/routine rehabilitation (see Table 4.1 for details). Studies combining CM therapies with pharmacotherapy/routine rehabilitation were required to use the same pharmacotherapy/routine rehabilitation in both the intervention and comparator groups;
- Comparators: Placebo, no treatment or pharmacotherapies or rehabilitation therapies that are recommended in international clinical practice guidelines (see Chapter 2 for details);
- Outcome measures: Studies reported at least one of the pre-specified outcome measures (Table 4.2).

Exclusion Criteria

Studies to be excluded in our systematic analyses are retrospective studies, epidemiological studies and studies designed as not using CM therapies to be the test therapy e.g. comparing CM therapy to other CM therapies, or CM combined with any of other therapies versus CM therapy.

- Participants: Any case of spasticity caused by another clinical condition, such as multiple sclerosis, traumatic brain and spinal cord injuries, etc.;

Table 4.2 Pre-specified Outcomes

Outcome Categories	Outcome Measures	Scoring
Motor function	1. Fugl-Meyer Assessment (FMA) – motor function	1. Up to 100 points; higher is better
	2. Fugl-Meyer Assessment (FMA) – upper limbs motor function	2. Up to 66 points; higher is better
	3. Fugl-Meyer Assessment (FMA) – lower limbs motor function	3. Up to 34 points; higher is better
Spasticity score	1. Ashworth Scale (AS)	1. 5 grades from 0–4; lower is better
	2. Modified Ashworth Scale (MAS)	2. 6 grades (0, 1, 1+, 2, 3, 4); lower is better
Activities of daily living	1. BI/MBI	1. Up to 100 points; higher is better
Adverse events	Number and type of adverse events	

Abbreviations: BI, Barthel index; MBI, modified Barthel index.

- Interventions: Any intervention other than those considered to be CM therapies;
- Comparators: Chinese medicine therapies and treatments other than those recommended in clinical practice guidelines;
- Outcome measures: Other outcome measures not outlined in Table 4.2.

Outcomes

Included outcomes were determined after consultation with the content expert advisory panel (CEAP) which was convened for this book. Outcomes of effect included known measures in post-stroke spasticity research (Table 4.2).

Ashworth Scale and Modified Ashworth Scale

The Ashworth scale was originally developed to assess the efficacy of an anti-spastic drug in patients suffering from multiple sclerosis.[4] The

Table 4.3 Grades of the Modified Ashworth Scale

Grade	Description
0	No increase in muscle tone.
1	Slight increase in muscle tone, manifested by a catch and release, or by minimal resistance at the end of the range of motion when the affected part(s) is moved in flexion or extension.
1+	Slight increase in muscle tone, manifested by a catch followed by minimal resistance throughout the remainder (less than half) of the range of movement (ROM).
2	More marked increase in muscle tone through most of the ROM, but affected part(s) easily moved.
3	Considerable increase in muscle tone; passive movement difficult.
4	Affected part(s) rigid in flexion or extension.

scale is used to assign a subjective rating of the amount of resistance or tone perceived by the examiner as a limb is moved through its full range of motion. The original Ashworth scale (AS) consisted of five grades, from 0 to 4. In 1987, Bohannon and Smith added one grade (1+) and revised the wording of the scale, renaming it the modified Ashworth scale (MAS) (see Table 4.3) in an attempt to make the scale more sensitive.[5–7] Changes to wording incorporated approximations of how much resistance was perceived and at what point during the motion resistance was felt.

The MAS has gained widespread clinical acceptance. It is routinely used to assess spasticity, and indeed is the current clinical standard.[8] However, there remains some questions as to whether the AS is a valid measure of spasticity. Currently there are no standardised testing procedures or guidelines for the use of the scale. While testing should be relatively brief, manipulation of the affected limb/joint may be uncomfortable for patients.

Fugl-Meyer Assessment of Motor Recovery After Stroke

The Fugl-Meyer Assessment (FMA) is a disease-specific impairment index designed to assess motor function, balance, sensation qualities and joint function in hemiplegic post-stroke patients.[9,10] The scale comprises five domains: (1) motor function (in the upper and lower extremities); (2) sensory function; (3) balance (both standing and sitting); (4) joint range of motion; and (5) joint pain. Items in the motor domain were derived from Twitchell's 1951 description of the natural history of motor recovery following stroke, which incorporates Brunnstrom's stages of motor recovery.[10]

Scale items are scored on the basis of ability to complete the item using a three-point ordinal scale where 0 = cannot perform, 1 = performs partially, and 2 = performs fully. The total possible scale score is 226. Points are divided among the domains as follows: 100 points for motor function (66 upper and 34 lower extremity); 24 points for sensation (light touch and position sense); 14 points for balance (6 sitting and 8 standing); 44 points for joint range of motion; and 44 points for joint pain. Classifications for impairment severity have been proposed based on FMA scores.[11,12]

It is not uncommon for the sections of the FMA to be administered separately. Administration of the entire test can be a lengthy process; it should take approximately 30–45 minutes to administer the total FMA. However, when the motor scale is administered on its own, it takes approximately 20 minutes. Assessments are completed by direct observation on a one-to-one basis and should be performed by a trained physical therapist.[10]

The FMA is widely used and internationally accepted. The motor assessment is grounded in well-defined, observable stages of motor recovery.[10] The FMA has been used as the gold standard against which the validity of other scales is assessed.

Barthel Index or Modified Barthel Index

The Barthel Index (BI) of activities of daily living (ADL) has been in use since 1965.[13] It was originally intended as a simple index of independence by which to quantify the ability of a patient with a neuromuscular or musculoskeletal disorder to care for him/herself (regardless of particular diagnostic designations). It is, perhaps, the most widely used measure of functional disability.

The BI is very simple, consisting of ten common ADL activities administered through direct observation. These are assessed for independence/dependence and scored via an arbitrary weighting system. Eight of the ten items represent activities related to personal care; the remaining two are related to mobility. The index yields a total score out of 100 — the higher the score, the greater the degree of functional independence.[13]

Based on the original version of the BI, a modified version (Modified Barthel Index — MBI) was introduced by Shah and Vanchay to increase the sensitivity of measurement.[14] This version of MBI assessed dependency using scores ranging from 0 (unable to perform task) to a maximum of 5, 10 or 15 (fully independent) for ten domains of functioning (activities): bowel control, bladder control, as well as help with grooming, toilet use, feeding, transfers, walking, dressing, climbing stairs and bathing.[14] The MBI achieved greater sensitivity and improved reliability than the original version, without causing additional difficulty or affecting the implementation time.[14] In addition, another MBI version was also adapted from the original BI scale, which covers the same ten domains but gives a maximum score of 20 (scores ranging from 0 to 2 or 3 for each activity).[15] However, there is a lack of agreement regarding the threshold for independence/dependence, and several different scoring systems are used, making comparisons across groups/studies more difficult.[3]

Risk of Bias Assessment

Risk of bias was assessed for RCTs using the Cochrane Collaboration's tool.[1] In clinical trials, bias can be categorised as selection bias, performance bias, detection bias, attrition bias and reporting bias. Each domain is assessed to determine whether the bias is at 'low', 'high', or 'unclear' risk. 'Low' risk of bias indicates that bias is unlikely, 'high' risk indicates plausible bias that seriously weakens confidence in the results and 'unclear' risk of bias indicates lack of information, or uncertainty, over potential bias and raises some doubt about the results. Risk of bias assessment was verified by two people and disagreement was resolved by discussion or consultation with a third person.

Risk of bias is categorised using the following six domains:

- Sequence generation: The method used to generate the allocation sequence is given in sufficient detail to allow an assessment of whether it should produce comparable groups. 'Low' risk of bias refers to a random number table or computer random generator. 'High' risk of bias includes studies that describe a non-random sequence generation such as odd or even date of birth or date of admission;
- Allocation concealment: The method used to conceal the allocation sequence is given in enough detail to determine whether intervention allocations could have been foreseen before or during enrolment. 'Low' risk of bias includes central randomisation or sealed envelopes and 'high' risk of bias includes open random sequence or date of birth, etc.
- Blinding of participants and personnel: Measures used to describe if the study participants and personnel are blind to the intervention received. In addition, information relating to whether the blinding was effective is also assessed. Studies that ensure blinding of participants and personnel are at 'low' risk of bias. If the study is not blind or incompletely blind it is at 'high' risk of bias.
- Blinding of outcome assessors: Measures used to describe if the outcome assessors are blind to knowledge of which intervention a participant received. In addition, information relating to whether the blinding was effective is also assessed. Studies that ensure blinding of outcome assessors are at 'low' risk of bias. If the study is not blind, or incompletely blind, it is at 'high' risk of bias.
- Incomplete outcome data: Completeness of outcome data for each main outcome, including drop-outs, exclusions from the analysis with numbers missing in each group, and reasons for drop-out or exclusions. Studies with 'low' risk of bias would include all outcome data; or if there is missing data, it is unlikely to relate to the true outcome or is balanced between groups. Studies at 'high' risk of bias would have unexplained missing data.

- Selective reporting: The study protocol is available, and the pre-specified outcomes are included in the report. Studies with a published protocol and which include all pre-specified outcomes in their report would be at 'low' risk of bias. Studies at 'high' risk of bias would not include all pre-specified outcomes or the outcome data may be reported incompletely.

Statistical Analyses

Frequency of CM syndromes, CHM formulas, herbs and acupuncture points reported in the included studies are presented using descriptive statistics. Chinese medicine syndromes reported in two or more studies were presented. The ten most frequently reported CHM formulas and 20 most frequently reported herbs presented were used in at least two studies, although for CHM formulas this was not always possible. The top ten acupuncture points used in two or more studies are presented, or as available. Where data was limited, reports of single CM syndromes or acupuncture points are provided as a guide for the reader.

Definitions of statistical tests and results are described in the glossary. Dichotomous data are reported as a risk ratio (RR) with 95% confidence interval (CI), and continuous data are reported as mean difference (MD) or standard mean difference (SMD) with 95% CI. For all analyses, RR, MD or SMD together with 95% CI were reported, as well as a formal test for heterogeneity using the I^2 statistic. An I^2 score greater than 50% was considered to indicate substantial heterogeneity.[1] Sensitivity analyses were undertaken to explore potential sources of heterogeneity, based on 'low' risk of bias for one of the risk of bias domains, namely sequence generation. Where possible and appropriate, planned subgroup analyses included duration of disease or treatment, CM syndromes, CM formulas and comparator type. Available case analysis with a random effects model was used in all analyses. The random effects model was used to take into account the clinical heterogeneity likely to be encountered within, and between, included studies, and the variation in treatment effects between included studies.

Assessment Using Grading of Recommendations Assessment, Development and Evaluation

The Grading of Recommendations Assessment, Development and Evaluation (GRADE) approach was used.[16] The GRADE approach summarises and rates the strength and certainty (quality) of evidence in systematic reviews using a structured process for presenting evidence summaries. The results are presented in summary of findings tables. The results provide an important overview for post-stroke spasticity outcomes.

A panel of experts was established to evaluate the certainty of evidence. The panel included the systematic review team, CM practitioners, integrative medicine experts, research methodologists and conventional medicine physicians. The experts were asked to rate the clinical importance of key interventions from CHM, acupuncture therapies and other CM therapies, as well as comparators and outcomes. Results were collated and based on the rating scores and subsequent discussion, and a consensus on the content for the summary of findings tables were achieved.

The certainty of evidence for each outcome was rated according to five factors outlined in the GRADE approach. The certainty of evidence may be rated based on:

- Limitations in study design (risk of bias);
- Inconsistency of results (unexplained heterogeneity);
- Indirectness of evidence (interventions, populations and outcomes important to the patients with the condition);
- Imprecision (uncertainty about the results);
- Publication bias (selective publication of studies).

These five factors are additive and a reduction in more than one factor will reduce the certainty of the evidence for that outcome. The GRADE approach also includes three domains that can be rated up, including large magnitude of an effect, dose-response gradient and effect of plausible residual confounding. However, these three domains relate to observational studies including cohort, case-control, before-after and time-series studies, etc. Grading of Recommendations Assessment, Development and Evaluation summaries in this book only include RCTs; therefore these three domains for rating up were not assessed.

Treatment recommendations can also be assessed using the GRADE approach, but due to the diverse nature of CM practice, treatment recommendations were not included with the summary of findings. Therefore, the reader is able to interpret the evidence with reference to the local practice environment. It should also be noted that the GRADE approach requires judgments about the certainty of evidence and some subjective assessment. However, the experience of the panel members suggests the judgments are reliable and transparent representations of the certainty of evidence.

The GRADE levels of evidence are grouped into four categories:

1. 'High' certainty evidence: Further research is very unlikely to change our confidence in the estimate of effect;
2. 'Moderate' certainty evidence: Further research is likely to have an important impact on our confidence in the estimate of effect and may change the estimate;
3. 'Low' certainty evidence: Further research is very likely to have an important impact on our confidence in the estimate of effect and is likely to change the estimate;
4. 'Very low' certainty evidence: Any estimate of effect is very uncertain.

References

1. Higgins J, Green S, eds. (2011) Cochrane Handbook for Systematic Reviews of Interventions Version 5.1.0. The Cochrane Collaboration. Available from: http://www.cochrane-handbook.org.
2. Duncan PW, Zorowitz R, Bates B, *et al.* (2005) Management of adult stroke rehabilitation care: A clinical practice guideline. *Stroke* **36(9):** e100–e143.
3. Robert WT, Norine CF, Norhayati H, *et al.* (2015) Evidence-based review of stroke rehabilitation, 17th ed. Available from: http://www.

ebrsr.com/sites/default/files/documents/executive-summary-srebr_final_16ed.pdf.
4. Ashworth B. (1964) Preliminary trial of carisoprodal in multiple sclerosis. *Practitioner* **192:** 540–542.
5. Bohannon RW, Smith MB. (1987) Interrater reliability of a modified Ashworth scale of muscle spasticity. *Phys Ther* **67(2):** 206–207.
6. Gregson JM, Leathley MJ, Moore AP, *et al.* (2000) Reliability of measurements of muscle tone and muscle power in stroke patients. *Age Ageing* **29(3):** 223–228.
7. Pandyan AD, Johnson GR, Price CI, *et al.* (1999) A review of the properties and limitations of the Ashworth and modified Ashworth Scales as measures of spasticity. *Clin Rehabil* **13(5):** 373–383.
8. van Wijck FM, Pandyan AD, Johnson GR, Barnes MP. (2001) Assessing motor deficits in neurological rehabilitation: Patterns of instrument usage. *Neurorehabil Neural Repair* **15(1):** 23–30.
9. Fugl-Meyer AR, Jaasko L, Leyman I, *et al.* (1975) The post-stroke hemiplegic patient. 1. A method for evaluation of physical performance. *Scand J Rehabil Med* **7(1):** 13–31.
10. Gladstone DJ, Danells CJ, Black SE. (2002) The Fugl-Meyer assessment of motor recovery after stroke: A critical review of its measurement properties. *Neurorehabil Neural Repair* **16(3):** 232–240.
11. Duncan PW, Goldstein LB, Horner RD, *et al.* (1994) Similar motor recovery of upper and lower extremities after stroke. *Stroke* **25(6):** 1181–1188.
12. Fugl-Meyer AR. (1980) Post-stroke hemiplegia assessment of physical properties. *Scand J Rehabil Med Suppl* **7:** 85–93.
13. Mahoney FI, Barthel DW. (1965) Functional evaluation: The Barthel index. *Md State Med J* **14:** 61–65.
14. Shah S, Vanclay F, Cooper B. (1989) Improving the sensitivity of the Barthel Index for stroke rehabilitation. *J Clin Epidemiol* **42:** 703–709.
15. Collin C, Wade DT, Davies S, Horne V. (1988) The Barthel ADL Index: A reliability study. *Int Disabil Stud* **10(2):** 61–63.
16. Schunemann H, Brozek J, Guyatt G, Oxman A, eds. (2013) GRADE handbook for grading quality of evidence and strength of recommendations. The GRADE Working Group. Available from: http://www.guidelinedevelopment.org/handbook/.

5

Clinical Evidence for Chinese Herbal Medicine

OVERVIEW

The clinical evidence for Chinese herbal medicine for post-stroke spasticity is evaluated in this chapter. Comprehensive searches in five English and four Chinese databases were conducted, identifying 22,597 citations, according to selection criteria. Sixty-two randomised controlled trials and nine non-controlled clinical studies are included in this chapter. The effects of oral, topical, and a combination of oral and topical Chinese herbal medicine therapies integrated with routine therapy and rehabilitation for post-stroke spasticity were evaluated in terms of spasticity severity, motor function of extremities and activity of daily living. Conclusions of the effects of Chinese herbal medicine for post-stroke spasticity could not be drawn based on the clinical evidence available due to a limitation in the number of included studies and their relatively poor methodological quality.

Introduction

Chinese herbal medicine (CHM) has been examined by many studies which have been published in scientific journals, both in China and internationally. A rigorous screening process was undertaken to identify clinical studies of CHM for the treatment of post-stroke spasticity. These studies included randomised controlled trials (RCTs), non-randomised controlled clinical trials (CCTs) and non-controlled studies. Data from RCTs and non-randomised controlled trials were evaluated for efficacy and safety. Non-controlled clinical studies were summarised for key information of relevant treatments.

Previous Systematic Reviews

Our search identified one systematic review on 10 RCTs published between 1990 and 2015 which evaluated the effects of the oral CHM formula *Shao yao gan cao tang* 芍药甘草汤 for post-stroke spasticity.[1] These RCTs were all conducted in China and involved 732 Chinese participants. Using a Jadad scale, the methodological quality of the included studies was scored 1 to 2.

In this review, the outcome measures were effective rate, Fugl-Meyer Assessment (FMA) and Barthel Index (BI). But the calculation methods of effective rate were not clearly defined. With regards to the safety of CHM, adverse events were described and calculated. Results of meta-analyses showed that oral *Shao yao gan cao tang* 芍药甘草汤 was beneficial for stroke patients with spasticity in terms of FMA (seven studies, mean difference (MD): 9.22 [6.31, 12.14]) and BI (four studies, MD: 7.11 [4.34, 9.89]). However, such meta-analyses did not separate studies of *Shao yao gan cao tang* 芍药甘草汤 versus routine care from studies of its use as an add-on to routine care.

Identification of Clinical Studies

Comprehensive searches of five English and four Chinese databases were conducted, with a total of 22,597 studies identified. According to our pre-defined selection criteria, 62 randomised controlled trials (H1 to H62) and nine non-controlled clinical studies (H63 to H71) were included in our analyses and presented in this chapter. Presentation of clinical evidence of CHM interventions was grouped based on the specific type of CHM therapy, including oral CHM, topical CHM, and the combination of oral and topical CHM.

Among the 62 RCTs, 27 studies evaluated the effects of oral CHM, 24 studies investigated topical CHM and the remaining 11 studies assessed the combination of oral plus topical CHM. Data of nine studies (H25, H29, H37, H42, H48, H54, H59–H61) could not be pooled in meta-analyses due to their variation in reporting outcome measures. The number of non-controlled clinical studies investigating the effects of oral, topical, and the combination of oral and topical CHM was seven, one and one respectively. One identified study with an intervention not commonly practised outside of China is not presented here (Fig. 5.1).

Oral Chinese Herbal Medicine

A total of 34 clinical studies evaluating the effects of oral CHM met our inclusion criteria. Among them, 27 studies are RCTs and seven are non-controlled studies. In this section, the RCTs were analysed for efficacy and safety while the non-controlled studies were summarised for key information.

Randomised Controlled Trials of Oral Chinese Herbal Medicine

Three comparison types were found in the 27 RCTs: one trial (H62) on oral CHM versus placebo; seven trials (H1, H20, H25, H30, H31, H35, H56) on oral CHM versus routine care or pharmacological therapies (i.e. oral baclofen or eperisone hydrochloride); and 18 trials (H2, H3, H5, H13, H14, H16, H17, H19, H28, H29, H32–H34, H37, H57–H60) investigated the add-on effects of oral CHM to routine pharmacological therapies or rehabilitation therapies. One study (H21) contained three groups (*Shao yao gan cao tang* 芍药甘草汤 plus rehabilitation therapies, versus rehabilitation therapies, versus baclofen plus rehabilitation therapies); this study was included in both comparisons for analyses.

All RCTs were conducted in outpatient or inpatient departments of hospitals in China. A total of 1,612 participants were included in these studies. Of the studies that reported mean age, the average was 61.6 years. More males than females were included (994 versus 589 respectively) among trials that reported information of gender. Of

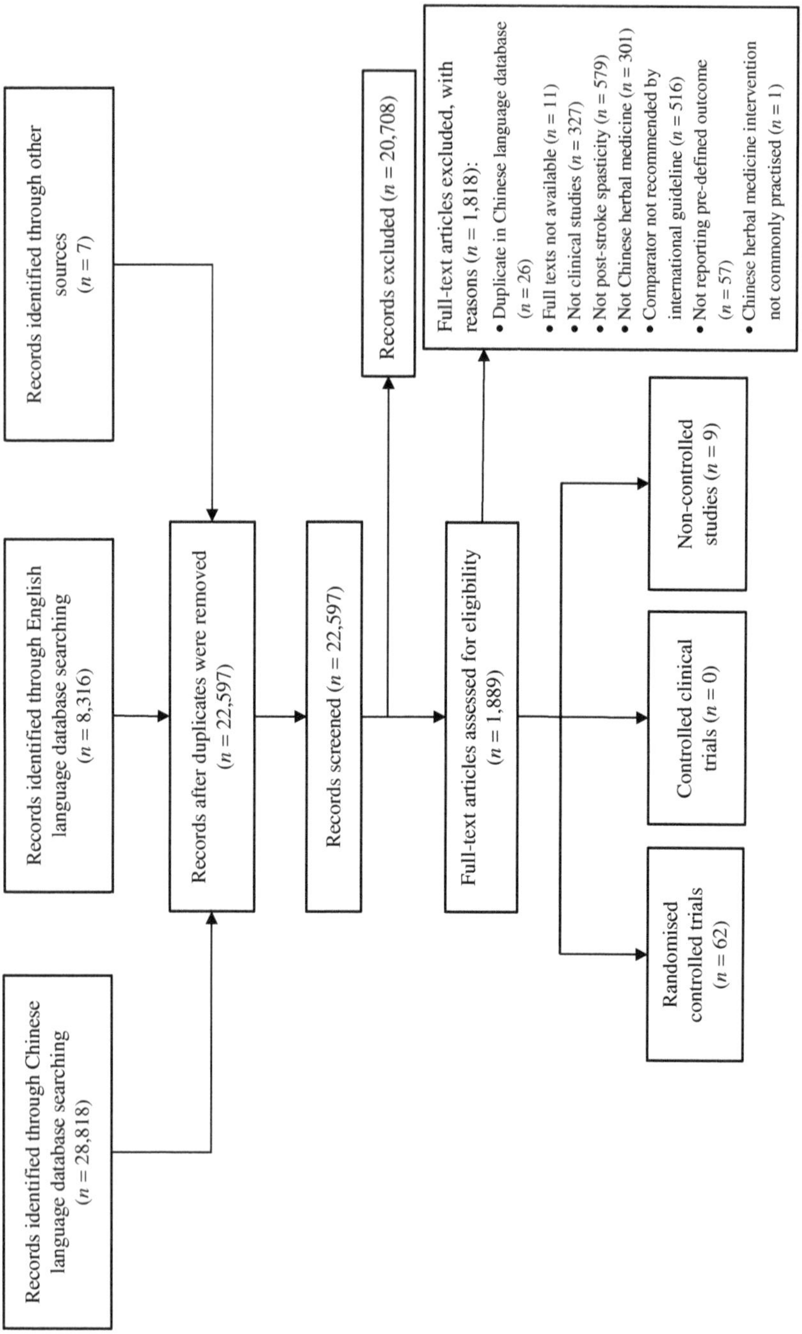

Fig. 5.1 Flowchart of study selection process: Chinese herbal medicine.

studies reporting the average post-stroke period, the average duration was 58.7 days. Two studies (H16, H19) used the Chinese medicine (CM) syndrome 'Wind, Phlegm and Blood stasis blocking meridians 风痰瘀血，痹阻脉络证' and '*yin* deficiency with Wind disturbing 阴虚风动' as inclusion criteria, while such a syndrome approach was not applied in any other study for inclusion or treatment.

The oral CHM formulas evaluated by the included studies varied considerably. For the administration of CHM decoction, the common approach among the included RCTs was to take 100–250 ml of oral CHM decoction twice a day for 14 to 56 days.

Three formulas were each evaluated in two studies: *Bu yang huan wu tang* 补阳还五汤 (H5, H33), *Gua lou gui zhi tang* 瓜蒌桂枝汤 (H14, H60) and *Shao yao gan cao tang* 芍药甘草汤 (H20, H21) (see Table 5.1).

The most frequently used herbs used in RCTs are presented in Table 5.2.

Risk of Bias Assessment

All included studies were described as RCTs. Six of them (H14, H25, H28, H34, H60, H62) applied appropriate methods for randomisation sequence generation and therefore were assessed as 'low' risk of bias

Table 5.1 Frequently Reported Oral Formulas in Randomised Controlled Trials

Most Common Formulas	No. of Studies	Ingredients
Bu yang huan wu tang 补阳还五汤	2 (H5, H33)	*Huang qi* 黄芪, *dang gui* 当归, *chi shao* 赤芍, *di long* 地龙, *chuan xiong* 川芎, *hong hua* 红花 and *tao ren* 桃仁
Gua lou gui zhi tang 瓜蒌桂枝汤	2 (H14, H60)	*Gua lou gen* 栝楼, *gui zhi* 桂枝, *shao yao* 芍药, *gan cao* 甘草, *sheng jiang* 生姜 and *da zao* 大枣
Shao yao gan cao tang 芍药甘草汤	2 (H20, H21)	*Shao yao* 芍药 and *gan cao* 甘草

Ingredients are referenced to the *Zhong Yi Fang Ji Da Ci Dian* 中医方剂大辞典 where available, or to the included study if not available. The use of some herbs may be restricted in some countries. Readers are advised to comply with relevant regulations.

Table 5.2 Frequently Used Oral Herbs in Randomised Controlled Trials

Most Common Herbs	Scientific Name	Frequency of Use
Bai shao 白芍	*Paeonia lactiflora* Pall.	20
Dang gui 当归	*Angelica sinensis* (Oliv.) Diels	16
Gan cao 甘草	*Glycyrrhiza uralensis* Fisch.	14
Di long 地龙	*Pheretima aspergillum* (E. Perrier)	15
Huang qi 黄芪	*Astragalus membranaceus* (Fisch.) Bge. var. *mongholicus* (Bge.) Hsiao	12
Chuan xiong 川芎	*Ligusticum chuanxiong* Hort.	10
Tao ren 桃仁	*Prunus Persica* (L.) Batsch	10
Shen jin cao 伸筋草	*Lycopodium japonicum* Thunb.	9
Hong hua 红花	*Carthamus tinctorius* L.	9
Ji xie teng 鸡血藤	*Spatholobus suberectus* Dunn	8
Sheng di huang 生地黄	*Regnabbua glutinosa* Libosch.	8
Gui zhi 桂枝	*Cinnamomum cassia* Presl.	7
Chi shao 赤芍	*Paeonia lactiflora* Pall.	7
Mu gua 木瓜	*Chaenomeles speciosa* (Sweet) Nakai	6
Quan xie 全蝎	*Buthus martensii* Karsch.	4
Shu di huang 熟地黄	*Regnabbua glutinosa* Libosch.	4
Shi hu 石斛	*Dendrobium nobile* Lindl.	4
Da zao 大枣	*Ziziphus jujube* Mill.	4
Niu xi 牛膝	*Achyranthes bidentata* Bl.	4

The use of some herbs may be restricted in some countries. Readers are advised to comply with relevant regulations.

for this domain; the other studies were assessed as 'unclear' risk due to lack of information. For the allocation concealment, three RCTs (H25, H60, H62) were assessed as 'low' risk of bias; the remaining studies were 'unclear' risk due to a lack of information. Blinding of participants and personnel was judged as 'low' risk of bias in only one study (H62), which applied a placebo control, while the others were assessed as 'high' risk of bias due to their design of comparing different treatments without making any effort for blinding. In terms of blinding of outcome assessors, all studies were assessed as 'unclear' risk of bias due to lack of information. With regard to incomplete outcome data, one study (H60) was assessed as 'high' risk of bias because no intention-to-treat analysis was applied for over 15% of the drop-outs. The other studies were judged as 'low' risk of bias. Two studies (H14, H37) were at 'high' risk of bias in selective reporting because they did not report all data on pre-defined outcome measures, while the others were assessed as 'unclear' risk of bias since their trial protocols were unavailable. Overall, the methodological quality of the included RCTs was low. Details of risk of bias assessment are available in Table 5.3.

Outcomes

The clinical assessment of spasticity severity mainly includes the neurological examination of muscle tone, motor power, reflexes and sensory level. The most frequently used validated scoring system is the Ashworth Scale (AS) or the Modified Ashworth Scale (MAS).[2,3] Considering the fact that post-stroke spasticity is often accompanied by other dysfunctions or may lead to secondary complications, in order to get an overall understanding of a patient's situation, a comprehensive assessment should preferably include motor function of extremities and quality of life, where FMA[4] and BI[5] are commonly used and reported in clinical trials for stroke patients. Therefore, we conducted meta-analyses on AS or MAS to assess the stiffness of muscles, FMA to measure

Table 5.3 Risk of Bias Assessment of Randomised Controlled Trials: Oral Chinese Herbal Medicine

Risk of Bias Domain	Low Risk *n* (%)	Unclear Risk *n* (%)	High Risk *n* (%)
Sequence generation	6 (22.2)	21 (77.8)	0 (0)
Allocation concealment	3 (11.1)	24 (88.9)	0 (0)
Blinding of participants	1 (3.7)	0 (0)	26 (96.3)
Blinding of personnel	1 (3.7)	0 (0)	26 (96.3)
Blinding of outcome assessors	0 (0)	100 (100.0)	0 (0)
Incomplete outcome data	26 (96.3)	0 (0)	1 (3.7)
Selective outcome reporting	0 (0)	25 (92.6)	2 (7.4)

motor function of extremities and BI for patients' daily activity for this book. The treatment effects of oral CHM were evaluated and presented below according to these pre-defined outcome measures.

Ashworth Scale or Modified Ashworth Scale

Upper limb

Meta-analysis of two RCTs (H21, H30) comparing oral CHM with routine pharmacotherapy/rehabilitation showed no significant difference (standardised mean difference (SMD): –0.31 [–0.63, 0.01], I^2 = 0%) (Table 5.4). When adding oral CHM to routine pharmacotherapy/rehabilitation, five studies (H13, H17, H19, H21, H34) reported data on the AS or MAS (upper limb). Meta-analysis of these five studies showed that the combination was more effective than routine pharmacotherapy/rehabilitation alone (SMD: –1.15 [–2.05, –0.25]), with high heterogeneity (I^2 = 94%) (Table 5.4). The source of high heterogeneity could not be detected through sensitivity analysis. One study (H62) compared oral CHM with placebo CHM, with no significant difference being detected in terms of MAS of the upper limb (MD: 0.08 [–0.21, 0.37]).

Lower limb

Comparing the combination of oral CHM and routine pharmacotherapy/rehabilitation with routine pharmacotherapy/rehabilitation alone, meta-analysis of six studies (H2, H3, H13, H19, H34, H57) showed that the combination was more effective for MAS (lower limb) (SMD: –1.10 [–1.85, –0.35]), but with high heterogeneity (I^2 = 89%) (Table 5.4). The source of high heterogeneity could not be detected through sensitivity analysis.

Non-specified

No significant difference was detected by meta-analysis of two studies (H35, H56) comparing oral CHM with pharmacotherapy/

Table 5.4 Meta-analyses Results of Oral Chinese Herbal Medicine at the End of Treatment

Comparison	Outcome	No. of Studies	No. of Participants	Effect Size (MD or SMD [95% CI])	I^2 %	Included Studies
Oral CHM versus pharmacotherapy and/or rehabilitation alone	AS or MAS (upper limb)	2	158	SMD: −0.31 [−0.63, 0.01]	0	H21, H30
	AS or MAS (non-specified region)	2	98	SMD: −0.24 [−0.76, 0.28]	39	H35, H56
	FMA (motor)	4	228	MD: 12.78 [8.11, 17.45]*	0	H1, H20, H35, H56
	BI	3	160	MD: 9.87 [5.04, 14.71]*	42	H20, H31, H56
Oral CHM as integrative medicine versus pharmacotherapy and/or rehabilitation therapies	AS or MAS (upper limb)	5	382	SMD: −1.15 [−2.05, −0.25]*	94	H13, H17, H19, H21, H34
	AS or MAS (lower limb)	6	334	SMD: −1.10 [−1.85, −0.35]*	89	H2, H3, H13, H19, H34, H57
	AS or MAS (non-specified)	2	135	SMD: −0.55 [−1.59, 0.50]	88	H5, H16
	FMA (motor)	6	416	MD: 8.80 [3.25, 14.35]*	85	H2, H3, H14, H16, H28, H32
	FMA (upper limb)	3	137	MD: 3.05 [0.17, 5.93]*	33	H5, H19, H57
	FMA (lower limb)	3	137	MD: 4.08 [2.47, 5.68]*	73	H5, H19, H57
	BI	9	553	MD: 8.47 [5.20, 11.74]*	78	H2, H5, H13, H14, H28, H32–H34, H57

*Statistically significant.

Abbreviations: AS – Ashworth Scale; BI – Barthel Index; CHM – Chinese herbal medicine; CI – confidence interval; FMA – Fugl-Meyer Assessment; MAS – Modified Ashworth Scale; MD – mean difference; SMD – standardised mean difference.

rehabilitation (SMD: −0.24 [−0.76, 0.28], I^2 = 39%) (Table 5.4). Another two studies (H5, H16) evaluated oral CHM as integrative medicine added to routine pharmacotherapy/rehabilitation, compared with pharmacotherapy/rehabilitation alone; there was also no significant difference (SMD: −0.55 [−1.59, 0.50], I^2 = 88%) (Table 5.4). The source of high heterogeneity could not be detected through sensitivity analysis.

Fugl-Meyer Assessment

Motor

Four studies (H1, H20, H35, H56) comparing oral CHM to routine pharmacotherapy and/or rehabilitation reported the score of FMA (motor function); the results showed that oral CHM was superior to routine pharmacotherapy and/or rehabilitation (MD: 12.78 [8.11, 17.45], I^2 = 0%) (Table 5.4). Six studies (H2, H3, H14, H16, H28, H32) evaluated the add-on effects of oral CHM to routine pharmacotherapy/rehabilitation alone. It was found that the combination was more effective (MD: 8.80 [3.25, 14.35]), though with high heterogeneity (I^2 = 85%) (Table 5.4).

Upper limb

Meta-analysis of three studies (H5, H19, H57) comparing the combination of oral CHM and routine pharmacotherapy/rehabilitation, to routine pharmacotherapy/rehabilitation alone, showed that the combination achieved greater effects (MD: 3.05 [0.17, 5.93], I^2 = 33%) (Table 5.4). It is worth noting that one study (H62) showed that oral CHM was more effective than placebo with regard to FMA (upper limb) (MD: 7.48 [0.37, 14.59]).

Lower limb

Three studies (H5, H19, H57) comparing the combination of oral CHM and routine pharmacotherapy/rehabilitation with routine pharmacotherapy/rehabilitation alone reported data on this outcome. Meta-analysis favoured the combination group (MD: 4.08 [2.47, 5.68], I^2 = 0%) (Table 5.4).

Barthel Index

Three studies (H20, H31, H56) that compared oral CHM with routine pharmacotherapy/rehabilitation reported data on BI. Meta-analysis showed that oral CHM was superior to routine pharmacotherapy/rehabilitation alone (MD: 9.87 [5.04, 14.71], I^2 = 42%) (Table 5.4). Nine studies (H2, H5, H13, H14, H28, H32–H34, H57) comparing the combination of oral CHM and routine pharmacotherapy/rehabilitation, to routine pharmacotherapy/rehabilitation alone, also reported data on this outcome. Meta-analysis showed that adding oral CHM to routine pharmacotherapy/rehabilitation was more effective than routine pharmacotherapy/rehabilitation alone (MD: 8.47 [5.20, 11.74]), with a substantial heterogeneity being detected (I^2 = 78%) (Table 5.4). But the source of high heterogeneity could not be detected through sensitivity analysis. One study (H62) compared oral CHM with placebo. No significant difference was shown between oral CHM and placebo (MD: –0.52 [–9.31, 8.27]).

Assessment Using Grading of Recommendations Assessment, Development and Evaluation

The overall certainty of clinical evidence of oral CHM compared to routine pharmacotherapy and oral CHM used as integrative therapy compared to routine pharmacotherapy/rehabilitation alone for post-stroke spasticity is low (Tables 5.5 and 5.6). The certainty of clinical evidence of oral CHM compared to placebo is moderate (Table 5.7); however, the small number of participants involved limits our confidence in the judgment of quality of evidence.

Frequently Reported Orally Used Herbs in Meta-analyses Showing Favourable Effect for Post-stroke Spasticity

The most frequently reported herbs from studies favouring the use of oral CHM for post-stroke spasticity were calculated and are presented in Table 5.8. Frequency is grouped according to outcome measures (MAS, FMA and BI).

Table 5.5 GRADE: Oral Chinese Herbal Medicine versus Routine Pharmacotherapy/ Rehabilitation for Post-stroke Spasticity

Outcomes	No. of Participants (Studies)	Certainty of the Evidence (GRADE)	Anticipated Absolute Effects	
			Risk with Pharmacotherapy	Risk Difference with Oral CHM (95% CI)
AS or MAS (upper limb)	158 (2 RCTs)	⊕⊕○○ LOW[a,b]	–	SMD **0.31 lower** (0.63 lower to 0.01 higher)
MAS (lower limb)	60 (1 RCT)	⊕⊕○○ LOW[a,b]	The mean MAS was **2.23.**	MD **0.67 lower** (1.00 lower to 0.34 lower)
FMA (motor)	228 (4 RCTs)	⊕⊕○○ LOW[a,b]	The mean FMA was **51.93.**	MD **12.78 higher** (8.11 higher to 17.45 higher)
FMA (upper limb)	60 (1 RCT)	⊕⊕○○ LOW[a,b]	The mean FMA was **25.03.**	MD **22.8 higher** (16.82 higher to 28.78 higher)
FMA (lower limb)	60 (1 RCT)	⊕⊕○○ LOW[a,b]	The mean FMA was **27.21.**	MD **14.59 higher** (10.53 higher to 18.65 higher)
BI	160 (3 RCTs)	⊕⊕○○ LOW[b,c]	The mean BI was **58.52.**	MD **9.87 higher** (5.04 higher to 14.71 higher)

The risk in the intervention group (and its 95% confidence interval) is based on the assumed risk in the comparison group and the **relative effect** of the intervention (and its 95% CI).

Abbreviations: AS – Ashworth Scale; BI – Barthel Index; CHM – Chinese herbal medicine; CI – confidence interval; FMA – Fugl-Meyer Assessment; MAS – Modified Ashworth Scale; MD – mean difference; RCT – randomised controlled trial; SMD – standardised mean difference.

Notes

[a]Lack of blinding of participants, personnel and assessors.
[b]Small sample size limits certainty of results.
[c]High statistical heterogeneity.

Study References

AS or MAS (upper limb): H21, H30
MAS (lower limb): H30
FMA (motor): H1, H20, H35, H56
FMA (upper limb): H30
FMA (lower limb): H30
BI: H20, H31, H56

Table 5.6 GRADE: Oral Chinese Herbal Medicine Used as Integrative Therapy Compared with Routine Pharmacotherapy/Rehabilitation Alone for Post-stroke Spasticity

Outcomes	No. of Participants (Studies)	Certainty of the Evidence (GRADE)	Anticipated Absolute Effects: Risk with Routine Pharmacotherapy and/or Rehabilitation	Anticipated Absolute Effects: Risk Difference with Oral CHM as Integrative (95% CI)
AS or MAS (upper limb)	382 (5 RCTs)	⊕⊕◯◯ LOW[a,b]	–	SMD **1.15 lower** (2.05 lower to 0.25 lower)
AS or MAS (lower limb)	334 (6 RCTs)	⊕⊕◯◯ LOW[a,b]	–	SMD **1.1 lower** (1.85 lower to 0.35 lower)
FMA (motor)	416 (6 RCTs)	⊕⊕◯◯ LOW[a,b]	The mean FMA was **65.10.**	MD **8.8 higher** (3.25 higher to 14.35 higher)
FMA (upper limb)	137 (3 RCTs)	⊕⊕◯◯ LOW[a,c]	The mean FMA was **29.46.**	MD **3.05 higher** (0.17 higher to 5.93 higher)
FMA (lower limb)	137 (3 RCTs)	⊕⊕◯◯ LOW[a,c]	The mean FMA was **21.91.**	MD **4.08 higher** (2.47 higher to 5.68 higher)
BI	553 (9 RCTs)	⊕⊕◯◯ LOW[a,b]	The mean BI was **53.36.**	MD **8.47 higher** (5.2 higher to 11.74 higher)

The risk in the intervention group (and its 95% confidence interval) is based on the assumed risk in the comparison group and the **relative effect** of the intervention (and its 95% CI).

Abbreviations: AS – Ashworth Scale; BI – Barthel Index; CHM – Chinese herbal medicine; CI – confidence interval; FMA – Fugl-Meyer Assessment; MAS – Modified Ashworth Scale; MD – mean difference; RCT – randomised controlled trial; SMD – standardised mean difference.

Notes

[a]Lack of blinding of participants, personnel and assessors.

[b]High statistical heterogeneity.

[c]Small sample size limits certainty of results.

Study References

AS or MAS (upper limb): H13, H17, H19, H21, H34

AS or MAS (lower limb): H2, H3, H13, H19, H34, H57

FMA (motor): H2, H3, H14, H16, H28, H32

FMA (upper limb): H5, H19, H57

FMA (lower limb): H5, H19, H57

BI: H2, H5, H13, H14, H28, H32–H34, H57

Table 5.7 GRADE: Oral Chinese Herbal Medicine versus Placebo for Post-stroke Spasticity

Outcomes	No. of Participants (Studies)	Certainty of the Evidence (GRADE)	Anticipated Absolute Effects: Risk with Placebo	Anticipated Absolute Effects: Risk Difference with Oral CHM (95% CI)
MAS (upper limb)	50 (1 RCT)	⊕⊕⊕◯ MODERATE[a]	The mean AS was **1.38.**	MD **0.08 higher** (0.21 lower to 0.37 higher)
FMA (upper limb)	50 (1 RCT)	⊕⊕⊕◯ MODERATE[a]	The mean FMA was **30.56.**	MD **7.48 higher** (0.37 higher to 14.59 higher)
BI	50 (1 RCT)	⊕⊕⊕◯ MODERATE[a]	The mean BI was **43.56.**	MD **0.52 lower** (9.31 lower to 8.27 higher)

The risk in the intervention group (and its 95% confidence interval) is based on the assumed risk in the comparison group and the **relative effect** of the intervention (and its 95% CI).

Abbreviations: BI – Barthel Index; CHM – Chinese herbal medicine; CI – confidence interval; FMA – Fugl-Meyer Assessment; MAS – Modified Ashworth Scale; MD – mean difference; RCT – randomised controlled trial; SMD – standardised mean difference.

Notes

[a]Small sample size limits certainty of results.

Study References

MAS (upper limb): H62

FMA (upper limb): H62

BI: H62

Non-controlled Clinical Studies of Oral Chinese Herbal Medicine

Seven non-controlled clinical studies (H63, H64–H68, H70) assessing oral CHM for post-stroke spasticity were identified through the search; four studies (H63, H64, H67, H68) were single-case reports and the other three (H65, H66, H70) were case series. A total of 112 participants were included in the seven studies.

Seven different formulas (*Shao yao gan cao tang* 芍药甘草汤, *Shu jin zhi jing tang* 舒筋止痉汤, *Gui zhi fu zi tang* 桂枝加附子汤, *Hua yu tong mai tang* 化瘀通脉汤, *Rou gan tong luo tang* and *Shu jin jie luan tang* 柔肝通络汤合舒筋解挛汤, *Zi ni yi qi yang yin fang* 自拟益气养阴方 and *Ju jing fang* 拘痉方) were used in the included studies; none of them had been evaluated in multiple studies. Among the

Table 5.8 Frequently Used Oral Herbs in Meta-analyses Showing Favourable Effect for Post-stroke Spasticity

Outcome Measure	No. of Meta-analyses	No. of Studies	Herbs	Scientific Name	Frequency of Use
AS or MAS	2	8	*Bai shao* 白芍	*Paeonia lactiflora* Pall.	4
			Dang gui 当归	*Angelica sinensis* (Oliv.) Diels	4
			Di long 地龙	*Pheretima aspergillum* (E. Perrier)	4
			Huang qi 黄芪	*Astragalus membranaceus* (Fisch.) Bge. var. *mongholicus* (Bge.) Hsiao	4
			Chuan xiong 川芎	*Ligusticum chuangxiong* Hort.	3
			Gan cao 甘草	*Glycyrrhiza uralensis* Fisch.	3
			Shan zhu yu 山茱萸	*Cornus officinalis* Sieb. Et Zucc.	3
			Shen jin cao 伸筋草	*Lycopodium japonicum* Thunb.	3
			Sheng di huang 生地黄	*Regnabbua glutinosa* Libosch.	3
FMA	3	10	*Bai shao* 白芍	*Paeonia lactiflora* Pall.	6
			Dang gui 当归	*Angelica sinensis* (Oliv.) Diels	4
			Gan cao 甘草	*Glycyrrhiza uralensis* Fisch.	4
			Di long 地龙	*Pheretima aspergillum* (E. Perrier)	3
			Gui zhi 桂枝	*Cinnamomum cassia* Presl.	3

(*Continued*)

Table 5.8 (*Continued*)

Outcome Measure	No. of Meta-analyses	No. of Studies	Herbs	Scientific Name	Frequency of Use
			Huang qi 黄芪	*Astragalus membranaceus* (Fisch.) Bge. var. *mongholicus* (Bge.) Hsiao	3
			Ji xue teng 鸡血藤	*Spatholobus suberectus* Dunn	3
			Mu guo 木瓜	*Chaenomeles speciosa* (Sweet) Nakai	3
			Shen jin cao 伸筋草	*Lycopodium japonicum* Thunb.	3
			Tian ma 天麻	*Gastrodia elata* Bl.	3
BI	1	9	*Bai shao* 白芍	*Paeonia lactiflora* Pall.	7
			Dang gui 当归	*Angelica sinensis* (Oliv.) Diels	4
			Di long 地龙	*Pheretima aspergillum* (E. Perrier)	4
			Gan cao 甘草	*Glycyrrhiza uralensis* Fisch.	4
			Huang qi 黄芪	*Astragalus membranaceus* (Fisch.) Bge. var. *mongholicus* (Bge.) Hsiao	4
			Shen jin cao 伸筋草	*Lycopodium japonicum* Thunb.	3

Abbreviations: AS – Ashworth Scale; BI – Barthel Index; FMA – Fugl-Meyer Assessment; MAS – Modified Ashworth Scale.

reported ingredients, *bai shao* 白芍 was the most frequently used herb.

Two case series studies (H65, H70) recruited patients with post-stroke spasticity in the upper or lower limbs. The other study (H66) did not detail such information. The location of spasticity in the patient of one single case report (H63) was in the upper limb, while another one (H67) was in both the upper and lower limbs, and the other two studies (H64, H68) were in the lower limbs. Two studies (H65, H70) reported changes of spasticity with MAS and the Composite Spasticity Index. One study (H66) reported improvement in effective rate without detailed information. The remaining four studies (H63, H64, H67, H68) reported symptom improvement. All these seven studies concluded that oral CHM was effective for post-stroke spasticity. However, the effects were not compared to any control method. Adverse events were not reported by any of these studies.

Topical Chinese Herbal Medicine

A total of 25 clinical studies, including 24 RCTs and one non-controlled clinical study, evaluating the effects of topical CHM were identified using our inclusion criteria. In this section, the RCTs were analysed for efficacy and safety, while the key information from the non-controlled clinical study was summarised.

Randomised Controlled Trials of Topical Chinese Herbal Medicine

A total of 24 RCTs evaluated the efficacy and safety of topical CHM. There were four studies (H4, H15, H27, H50) comparing topical CHM with pharmacological therapies (i.e. oral baclofen or eperisone hydrochloride) or rehabilitation therapies, and 20 trials (H7, H18, H23, H24, H26, H36, H39, H41–H49, H51–H54) investigated the add-on effects of topical CHM to routine pharmacological therapies or rehabilitation therapies.

All studies were conducted in Chinese populations, from the inpatient or outpatient departments in hospitals in China. A total of 2,057 participants were included in these studies. Of the studies that reported mean age, the average was 62.1 years. More males were included than females (1,175 and 883, respectively) among trials that reported gender of participants. Of studies reporting the average post-stroke period, the average duration was 48.9 days. Chinese medicine syndrome was not applied in any of the included studies for diagnosis or treatment.

The topical CHM formulas varied across the included RCTs. For CHM topical application, the administration method was to apply topical CHM paste once, to three times per day for 15 to 80 days among the included RCTs. Only one formula, *Shu jin huo luo xi ji* 舒筋活络洗剂, was reported in multiple studies (H23, H24). The ingredients of this formula were *huang qi* 黄芪, *dang gui* 当归, *dang shen* 党参, *tao ren* 桃仁, *hong hua* 红花, *chuan xiong* 川芎, *su mu* 苏木, *sang zhi* 桑枝, *shen jin cao* 伸筋草, *ji xie teng* 鸡血藤, *mu gua* 木瓜, *wei ling xian* 威灵仙, *dan shen* 丹参 and *ma qian zi* 马钱子. Other studies all used different named formulas or unnamed formulas.

Moreover, we calculated the herbs reported among the included trials. The top 20 most frequently used ones are presented in Table 5.9.

Risk of Bias Assessment

All included studies were described as RCTs; seven of them (H18, H23, H24, H27, H44, H46, H49) applied appropriate methods for randomisation sequence generation and therefore were assessed as 'low' risk of bias for this domain; the other studies were assessed as 'unclear' risk due to insufficient information. For the allocation concealment, all RCTs were assessed as 'unclear' risk due to lack of information. Blinding of participants and personnel was judged as 'high' risk of bias in all the included RCTs because of their design of comparing different treatments without any effort of blinding. In terms of blinding of outcome assessors, all were assessed as 'unclear' risk of bias since they did not report blinding of assessors. With regard to incomplete outcome data, all included RCTs were judged as 'low' risk of bias. All studies were assessed as 'unclear' risk of bias because their trial protocols were unavailable. Overall, the methodological quality of the included RCTs was low, preventing us from drawing any firm conclusion on the effects of topical CHM for post-stroke spasticity. A summary of the details of risk of bias assessment is available in Table 5.10.

Table 5.9 Frequently Used Topical Herbs in Randomised Controlled Trials

Most Common Herbs	Scientific Name	Frequency of Use
Hong hua 红花	*Carthamus tinctorius* L.	18
Shen jin cao 伸筋草	*Lycopodium japonicum* Thunb.	12
Mu gua 木瓜	*Chaenomeles speciosa* (Sweet) Nakai	12
Dang gui 当归	*Angelica sinensis* (Oliv.) Diels	12
Chuan xiong 川芎	*Ligusticum chuanxiong* Hort.	10
Bai shao 白芍	*Paeonia lactiflora* Pall.	9
Gui zhi 桂枝	*Cinnamomum cassia* Presl.	9
Dan shen 丹参	*Salvia miltiorrhiza* Bge.	9
Su mu 苏木	*Caesalpinia sappan* L.	7
Di long 地龙	*Pheretima aspergillum* (E. Perrier)	7
Sang zhi 桑枝	*Morus alba* L.	6
Ji xie teng 鸡血藤	*Spatholobus suberectus* Dunn	6
Tou gu cao 透骨草	Herba Clematidis Intricatae	6
Wei ling xian 威灵仙	*Clematis chinensis* Osbeck.	5
Mo yao 没药	*Commiphora myrrha* Engl.	5
Ru xiang 乳香	*Boswellia carterii* Birdw.	5
Ai ye 艾叶	*Artemisia argyi* Lévl. et Vant.	5
Gan cao 甘草	*Glycyrrhiza uralensis* Fisch.	5
Tao ren 桃仁	*Prunus Persica* (L.) Batsch	5
Huang qi 黄芪	*Astragalus membranaceus* (Fisch.) Bge. var. *mongholicus* (Bge.) Hsiao	5

Outcomes

Ashworth Scale or Modified Ashworth Scale

Upper limb

The AS or MAS (upper limb) was reported by two RCTs (H15, H27) comparing topical CHM to routine pharmacotherapy/rehabilitation. Meta-analysis did not find any significant difference between topical CHM and routine pharmacotherapy/rehabilitation (SMD: −0.11 [−0.46, 0.24], $I^2 = 0\%$) (Table 5.11).

Table 5.10 Risk of Bias Assessment of Randomised Controlled Trials: Topical Chinese Herbal Medicine

Risk of Bias Domain	Low Risk *n* (%)	Unclear Risk *n* (%)	High Risk *n* (%)
Sequence generation	7 (28)	17 (72)	0 (0)
Allocation concealment	0 (0)	24 (100)	0 (0)
Blinding of participants	0 (0)	0 (0)	24 (100)
Blinding of personnel	0 (0)	0 (0)	24 (100)
Blinding of outcome assessors	0 (0)	24 (100)	0 (0)
Incomplete outcome data	24 (100)	0 (0)	0 (0)
Selective outcome reporting	0 (0)	24 (100)	0 (0)

Comparing the combination of topical CHM and routine pharmacotherapy/rehabilitation to routine pharmacotherapy/rehabilitation alone, seven studies (H26, H39, H43–H46, H49) reported data on the MAS (upper limb). Although meta-analysis of these studies showed that the combination was more effective than routine pharmacotherapy and/or rehabilitation alone (SMD: –0.97 [–1.37, –0.57]), the heterogeneity was high (I^2 = 76%) (Table 5.11). Heterogeneity was reduced to 0% when only studies assessed as low risk of bias in random sequence generation (H44, H46, H49) were included in sensitivity analysis.

Lower limb

No significant difference was found between topical CHM and routine pharmacotherapy/rehabilitation by meta-analysis of two studies (H4, H27) (SMD: –0.28 [–0.97, 0.40]) with substantial heterogeneity (I^2 = 75%) (Table 5.11). Comparing the combination of topical CHM and routine pharmacotherapy/rehabilitation to routine rehabilitation alone, six studies (H23, H26, H39, H43, H44, H46) reported data on the AS or MAS (lower limb). Meta-analysis of these studies showed that the combination was more effective than routine pharmacotherapy/rehabilitation alone (SMD: –0.82 [–1.15, –0.48], I^2 = 59%) (Table 5.11).

Table 5.11 Meta-analyses Results of Topical Chinese Herbal Medicine (at the End of Treatment)

Comparison	Outcome	No. of Studies	No. of Participants	Effect Size (MD or SMD [95% CI])	I^2 (%)	Included Studies
Topical CHM versus pharmaco-therapy/rehabilitation	AS or MAS (upper limb)	2	124	SMD: −0.11 [−0.46, 0.24]	0	H15, H27
	AS or MAS (lower limb)	2	140	SMD: −0.28 [−0.97, 0.40]	75	H4, H27
	FMA (upper limb)	2	120	MD: −2.69 [−3.51, −1.87]	0	H27, H51
	BI	2	120	MD: 5.06 [−6.66, 16.78]	90	H27, H50
Topical CHM used as integrative medicine versus pharmaco-therapy/rehabilitation	AS or MAS (upper limb)	7	475	SMD: −0.97 [−1.37, −0.57]*	76	H26, H39, H43–H46, H49
	AS or MAS (lower limb)	6	398	SMD: −0.82 [−1.15, −0.48]*	59	H23, H26, H39, H43, H44, H46
	AS or MAS (non-specified)	5	326	SMD: −0.99 [−1.99, 0.00]	94	H7, H18, H36, H42, H54
	FMA (motor)	4	326	MD: 11.89 [8.93, 14.85]*	12	H36, H48, H51, H54
	FMA (upper limb)	2	87	MD: 7.03 [3.12, 10.95]*	29	H24, H45
	BI	7	580	MD: 19.64 [14.73, 24.55]*	88	H26, H39, H43, H45, H51, H52, H54

*Statistically significant.

Abbreviations: AS – Ashworth Scale; BI – Barthel Index; CHM – Chinese herbal medicine; CI – confidence interval; FMA – Fugl-Meyer Assessment; MAS – Modified Ashworth Scale; MD – mean difference; SMD – standardised mean difference.

Non-specified

Five studies (H7, H18, H36, H42, H54) compared oral CHM as integrative medicine added to routine pharmacotherapy and/or rehabilitation with pharmacotherapy and/or rehabilitation alone; there was no significant difference between groups (SMD –0.99 [–1.99, 0.00]), with high heterogeneity (I^2 = 94%) (Table 5.11). The source of high heterogeneity could not be detected through sensitivity analysis.

Fugl-Meyer Assessment

Motor

Four studies (H36, H48, H51, H54) which compared the combination of topical CHM and routine pharmacotherapy/rehabilitation, to routine pharmacotherapy/rehabilitation alone, reported FMA (motor function). It was found that the combination was more effective than routine pharmacotherapy/rehabilitation alone (MD: 11.89 [8.93, 14.85], I^2 = 12%) (Table 5.11).

Upper limb

Two studies (H27, H50) compared the efficacy of topical CHM to that of routine pharmacotherapy and/or routine therapy. The results showed that topical CHM was inferior to routine pharmacotherapy and/or routine therapy (MD: –2.69 [–3.51, –1.87], I^2 = 0%) (Table 5.11). Two studies (H24, H45) comparing the combination of topical CHM and routine pharmacotherapy/rehabilitation, with routine pharmacotherapy/rehabilitation alone, reported data on this outcome. Meta-analysis showed that the combination achieved greater effects than routine pharmacotherapy/rehabilitation alone (MD: 7.03 [3.12, 10.95], I^2 = 29%) (Table 5.11).

Lower limb

One study (H27) compared the effects of topical CHM to routine pharmacotherapy. Topical CHM demonstrated better results for post-stroke spasticity than routine pharmacotherapy (MD: 3.70 [3.00, 4.40]). Only one study (H52) comparing the combination of topical CHM and rehabilitation to rehabilitation alone, reported data on this outcome. The results favoured the combination group (MD: 36.64 [31.21, 42.07]).

Barthel Index

Two studies (H27, H50) which compared topical CHM to routine pharmacotherapy/rehabilitation reported data on BI. Meta-analysis failed to show a significant difference between topical CHM and routine pharmacotherapy/rehabilitation (MD: 5.06 [–6.66, 16.78], $I^2 = 90\%$) (Table 5.11).

Seven studies (H26, H39, H43, H45, H51, H52, H54) comparing the combination of topical CHM and routine pharmacotherapy and/or rehabilitation, to routine pharmacotherapy and/or rehabilitation alone, also reported data on this outcome. Meta-analysis showed that adding topical CHM to routine pharmacotherapy/rehabilitation was more effective than routine pharmacotherapy/rehabilitation alone (MD: 19.64 [14.73, 24.55]), with considerable heterogeneity being detected ($I^2 = 98\%$) (Table 5.11). However, the source of high heterogeneity could not be detected through sensitivity analysis.

Assessment Using Grading of Recommendations Assessment, Development and Evaluation

The overall certainty of clinical evidence of topical CHM compared to routine pharmacotherapy and topical CHM used as integrative therapy for post-stroke spasticity is low (Tables 5.12 and 5.13). It is noted that there was moderate certainty of evidence to support using topical CHM as integrative medicine, compared to routine pharmacotherapy/rehabilitation, for reducing lower limb spasticity (assessed by AS or MAS). All other evidence was of very low to low certainty.

Table 5.12 GRADE: Topical Chinese Herbal Medicine versus Routine Pharmacotherapy/Rehabilitation

Outcomes	No. of Participants (Studies)	Certainty of the Evidence (GRADE)	Anticipated Absolute Effects: Risk with Pharmacotherapy and/or Rehabilitation	Anticipated Absolute Effects: Risk Difference with Topical CHM (95% CI)
AS or MAS (upper limb)	124 (2 RCTs)	⊕⊕○○ LOW[a,b]	–	SMD **0.11 lower** (0.46 lower to 0.24 higher)
AS or MAS (lower limb)	140 (2 RCTs)	⊕○○○ VERY LOW[a,b,c]	–	SMD **0.28 lower** (0.69 lower to 0.32 higher)
FMA (upper limb)	120 (2 RCTs)	⊕⊕○○ LOW[a,b]	The mean FMA was **56.07.**	MD **2.69 lower** (3.51 lower to 1.87 lower)
FMA (lower limb)	60 (1 RCT)	⊕⊕○○ LOW[a,b]	The mean FMA was **61.95.**	MD **3.70 higher** (3.00 higher to 4.40 higher)
BI	120 (2 RCTs)	⊕○○○ VERY LOW[a,b,c]	The mean BI was **74.38.**	MD **5.06 higher** (6.66 lower to 16.78 higher)

The risk in the intervention group (and its 95% confidence interval) is based on the assumed risk in the comparison group and the **relative effect** of the intervention (and its 95% CI).

Abbreviations: AS – Ashworth Scale; BI – Barthel Index; CHM – Chinese herbal medicine; CI – confidence interval; FMA – Fugl-Meyer Assessment; MAS – Modified Ashworth Scale; MD – mean difference; RCT – randomised controlled trial; SMD – standardised mean difference.

Notes

[a]Lack of blinding of participants, personnel and assessors.

[b]Small sample size limits certainty of results.

[c]High statistical heterogeneity.

Study References

AS or MAS (upper limb): H15, H27

AS or MAS (lower limb): H4, H27

FMA (upper limb): H27, H50

FMA (lower limb): H27

BI: H27, H50

Table 5.13 GRADE: Topical Chinese Herbal Medicine as Integrative Therapy versus Routine Pharmacotherapy/Rehabilitation

Outcomes	No. of Participants (Studies)	Certainty of the Evidence (GRADE)	Anticipated Absolute Effects: Risk with Pharmacotherapy and/or Rehabilitation	Anticipated Absolute Effects: Risk Difference with Topical CHM as Integrative Therapy (95% CI)
AS or MAS (upper limb)	475 (7 RCTs)	⊕⊕◯◯ LOW[a,b]	–	SMD **0.97 lower** (1.37 lower to 0.57 lower)
AS or MAS (lower limb)	398 (6 RCTs)	⊕⊕⊕◯ MODERATE[a,b]	–	SMD **0.82 lower** (1.15 lower to 0.48 lower)
FMA (motor)	326 (4 RCTs)	⊕⊕⊕◯ MODERATE[a]	The mean FMA was **46.50**.	MD **11.89 higher** (8.93 higher to 14.85 higher)
FMA (upper limb)	87 (2 RCTs)	⊕⊕◯◯ LOW[a,c]	The mean FMA was **24.25**.	MD **7.03 higher** (3.12 higher to 10.95 higher)
FMA (lower limb)	80 (1 RCT)	⊕⊕◯◯ LOW[a,c]	The mean FMA was **51.72**.	MD **36.64 higher** (31.21 higher to 40.07 higher)
BI	580 (7 RCTs)	⊕⊕◯◯ LOW[a,b]	The mean BI was **53.78**.	MD **19.64 higher** (14.73 higher to 24.55 higher)

The risk in the intervention group (and its 95% confidence interval) is based on the assumed risk in the comparison group and the **relative effect** of the intervention (and its 95% CI).

Abbreviations: AS – Ashworth Scale; BI – Barthel Index; CHM – Chinese herbal medicine; CI – confidence interval; FMA – Fugl-Meyer Assessment; MAS – Modified Ashworth Scale; MD – mean difference; RCT – randomised controlled trial; SMD – standardised mean difference.

Notes

[a]Lack of blinding of participants, personnel and assessors.

[b]High statistical heterogeneity.

[c]Small sample size limits certainty of results.

Study References

AS or MAS (upper limb): H26, H39, H43–H46, H49

AS or MAS (lower limb): H23, H26, H39, H43, H44, H46

FMA (motor): H36, H48, H51, H54

FMA (upper limb): H24, H45

FMA (lower limb): H52

BI: H26, H39, H43, H45, H51, H52, H54

Frequently Used Topical Herbs in Meta-analyses Showing Favourable Effect for Post-stroke Spasticity

The most frequently reported herbs from studies favouring integration of topical CHM for post-stroke spasticity were calculated and are presented in Table 5.14. Frequency is grouped according to outcome measures (MAS, FMA and BI). These herbs are similar to those found from oral CHM studies.

Table 5.14 Frequently Reported Topically Used Herbs in Meta-analyses Showing Favourable Effect for Post-stroke Spasticity

Outcome Measure	No. of Meta-analyses	No. of Studies	Herbs	Scientific Name	Frequency of Use
MAS	2	8	*Hong hua* 红花	*Carthamus tinctorius* L.	6
			Chuan xiong 川芎	*Ligusticum chuangxiong* Hort.	5
			Dang gui 当归	*Angelica sinensis* (Oliv.) Diels	5
			Bai shao 白芍	*Paeonia lactiflora* Pall.	4
			Mu guo 木瓜	*Chaenomeles speciosa* (Sweet) Nakai	4
			Shen jin cao 伸筋草	*Lycopodium japonicum* Thunb.	4
FMA	3	6	*Hong hua* 红花	*Carthamus tinctorius* L.	6
			Dang gui 当归	*Angelica sinensis* (Oliv.) Diels	4
			Chuan xiong 川芎	*Ligusticum chuangxiong* Hort.	3
			Dan shen 丹参	*Salvia miltiorrhiza* Bge.	3
			Di long 地龙	*Pheretima aspergillum* (E. Perrier)	3
			Gui zhi 桂枝	*Cinnamomum cassia* Presl.	3
			Ji xue teng 鸡血藤	*Spatholobus suberectus* Dunn	3
			Mu guo 木瓜	*Chaenomeles speciosa* (Sweet) Nakai	3
			Sang zhi 桑枝	*Morus alba* L.	3
			Shen jin cao 伸筋草	*Lycopodium japonicum* Thunb.	3
BI	1	7	*Dang gui* 当归	*Angelica sinensis* (Oliv.) Diels	5
			Di long 地龙	*Pheretima aspergillum* (E. Perrier)	5
			Hong hua 红花	*Carthamus tinctorius* L.	5
			Bai shao 白芍	*Paeonia lactiflora* Pall.	4
			Chuan xiong 川芎	*Ligusticum chuangxiong* Hort.	4
			Dan shen 丹参	*Salvia miltiorrhiza* Bge.	4

Non-controlled Clinical Studies of Topical Chinese Herbal Medicine

One case series (H71) which assessed topical CHM for post-stroke spasticity, was identified through the search. A total of 57 participants were included in the study and treated with fumigation of *Ju jing fang* (拘痉方), which included the ingredients *huang qi* 黄芪, *ji xie teng* 鸡血藤, *bai shao* 白芍, *gan cao* 甘草, *gu sui gu* 骨碎补, *mu gua* 木瓜, *dang gui* 当归, *shen jin cao* 伸筋草, *tou gu cao* 透骨草 and *hong hua* 红花. This study recruited patients with post-stroke spasticity in upper or lower limbs. The author of this study concluded that topical CHM was effective for post-stroke spasticity. However, the effects were not compared to any control method. Adverse events were not reported.

Oral plus Topical Chinese Herbal Medicine for Post-stroke Spasticity

A total of 12 clinical studies evaluating the effects of oral plus topical CHM met our inclusion criteria, including 11 RCTs and one non-controlled clinical study. In this section, the RCTs were analysed for efficacy and safety while the non-controlled clinical study was summarised for key information.

Randomised Controlled Trials of Oral plus Topical Chinese Herbal Medicine

A total of 11 RCTs evaluated the efficacy and safety of oral plus topical CHM. Two studies (H11, H12) compared oral plus topical CHM to routine care or pharmacological therapies (i.e. oral baclofen or tizanidine) and seven trials (H6, H9, H10, H22, H38, H40, H55) investigated the add-on effects of oral plus topical CHM to routine care (pharmacological therapies) or rehabilitation therapies. Two studies (H8, H61) were three-armed studies which contained both routine care (pharmacological therapies) and rehabilitation therapies as comparators.

All RCTs were conducted in Chinese populations, in outpatient or inpatient departments of hospitals. A total of 1,063 participants were included in these studies. Of the studies that reported mean age, the average was 54.8 years. More males were included than females (545 and 367, respectively) among trials that reported gender of participants. Of the studies that reported post-stroke period, the average duration was 37.1 days. Chinese medicine syndrome approach was not used in any of the included studies for diagnosis or treatment.

The oral and topical CHM formulas varied in the included RCTs. For CHM decoction, the administration method was to apply 100–150 ml of the oral CHM formulas once to twice per day for 28 to 30 days among the included RCTs. As for the topical CHM, it was applied once to twice per day for a similar duration of around 30 days.

The following formulas were reported in five and two studies, respectively: *Jie jing he ji* 解痉合剂 (H6, H8–H10, H61) and *Jie jing ke li* 解痉颗粒 (H11, H12) (Table 5.15). Moreover, we calculated the herbs reported among the included trials. Only nine herbs had been used by multiple studies; they are presented in Table 5.16.

Table 5.15 Frequently Reported Formulas Applied Orally and Topically in Randomised Controlled Trials

Most Common Formulas	No. of Studies	Admission Methods	Ingredients
Jie jing he ji 解痉合剂	5	Oral and topical	*Bai shao* 白芍, *gan cao* 甘草, *wang jiang nan* 望江南, *mu gua* 木瓜, *quan xie* 全蝎, *dan shen* 丹参 and *huang jiu* 黄酒
Jie jing ke li 解痉颗粒	2	Oral	*Shu di huang* 熟地黄, *bai shao* 白芍, *dang gui* 当归, *mu gua* 木瓜, *ji xie teng* 鸡血藤, *quan xie* 全蝎, *niu xi* 牛膝, *shen jin cao* 伸筋草 and *gan cao* 甘草

Ingredients are referenced to the *Zhong Yi Fang Ji Da Ci Dian* 中医方剂大辞典 where available, or to the included study if not available.

Table 5.16 Frequently Reported Herbs Used Both Orally and Topically in Randomised Controlled Trials

Most Common Herbs	Scientific Name	Frequency of Use
Bai shao 白芍	*Paeonia lactiflora* Pall.	6
Gan cao 甘草	*Glycyrrhiza uralensis* Fisch.	6
Mu gua 木瓜	*Chaenomeles speciosa* (Sweet) Nakai	5
Quan xie 全蝎	*Buthus martensii* Karsch	5
Wang jiang nan 望江南	*Cassia occidentalis* Linn	5
Dan shen 丹参	*Salvia miltiorrhiza* Bge.	5
Huang jiu 黄酒	N/A	4
Ru xiang 乳香	*Boswellia carterii* Birdw.	2
Mo yao 没药	*Commiphora myrrha* Engl.	2

Risk of Bias Assessment

All included studies were described as RCTs; five of them (H11, H12, H22, H38, H61) applied an appropriate method for randomisation sequence generation and therefore were assessed as 'low' risk of bias for this domain. One study (H9) was judged as 'high' risk of bias because it allocated patients based on the order of attendance; the other studies were assessed as 'unclear' risk due to insufficient information. For the allocation concealment, one RCT (H9) was assessed as 'high' risk of bias due to no concealment of allocation; the remaining studies were 'unclear' risk due to lack of information. Blinding of participants and personnel was judged as 'high' risk of bias due to their design of comparing different treatments without any effort at blinding. Similarly, in terms of blinding of outcome assessors, all included studies were assessed as 'unclear' risk of bias since they did not report blinding of assessors. In terms of incomplete outcome data, all RCTs were assessed as 'low' risk of bias. One study (H6) was at 'high' risk of bias in selective reporting due to reporting less outcomes (blood tests results) than what was described in its methods section; while the others were assessed as 'unclear' risk of bias because their trial protocols were unavailable. Overall, the methodological quality of the included RCTs was low, preventing us from drawing any firm

Table 5.17 Risk of Bias Assessment of Randomised Controlled Trials: Oral plus Topical Chinese Herbal Medicine

Risk of Bias Domain	Low Risk *n* (%)	Unclear Risk *n* (%)	High Risk *n* (%)
Sequence generation	5 (45.45)	5 (45.45)	1 (9.1)
Allocation concealment	0 (0)	10 (90.9)	1 (9.1)
Blinding of participants	0 (0)	0 (0)	11 (100)
Blinding of personnel	0 (0)	0 (0)	11 (100)
Blinding of outcome assessors	0 (0)	11 (100)	0 (0)
Incomplete outcome data	11 (100)	0 (0)	0 (0)
Selective outcome reporting	0 (0)	10 (90.9)	1 (9.1)

conclusion on the effects of oral plus topical CHM for post-stroke spasticity. Details of risk of bias assessment are available in Table 5.17 for a summary.

Outcomes

Ashworth Scale or Modified Ashworth Scale

Upper limb

Results of one study (H8) showed that there was no difference between oral plus topical CHM and routine pharmacotherapy (MD: –0.20 [–0.57, 0.17]). When adding oral plus topical CHM to routine pharmacotherapy/rehabilitation, meta-analysis of four studies (H8, H9, H22, H40) confirmed significant add-on effects of CHM (SMD: –0.69 [–0.91, –0.47], I^2 = 0%) (Table 5.18).

Lower limb

Results of one study (H8) showed that there was no difference between oral plus topical CHM and routine pharmacotherapy (MD: –0.13 [–0.43, 0.17]). Meta-analysis of five studies (H8, H9, H22, H38, H40) showed significant benefits of adding oral plus topical

CHM to routine pharmacotherapy/rehabilitation (SMD: –0.97 [–1.16, –0.77], I^2 = 0%) (Table 5.18).

Non-specified

Meta-analysis of two studies (H12, H61) showed that there was no significant difference between oral plus topical CHM and the routine therapies (SMD: –0.19 [–0.55, 0.16], I^2 = 43%) (Table 5.18). Two studies (H10, H61) evaluated oral plus topical CHM as integrative medicine added to routine pharmacotherapy/rehabilitation; the add-on effect was significant (SMD: –0.97 [–1.16, –0.77], I^2 = 0%) (Table 5.18).

Table 5.18 Meta-analyses Results of Oral Plus Topical Chinese Herbal Medicine (at the End of Treatment)

Comparison	Outcome	No. of Studies	No. of Participants	Effect size (MD or SMD [95% CI])	I^2 (%)	Included Studies
Oral plus topical CHM versus pharmacotherapy/rehabilitation	AS or MAS (non-specified)	2	235	SMD: –0.19 [–0.55, 0.16]	43	H12, H61
	FMA (motor)	4	445	MD: 4.20 [0.88, 7.52]*	38	H8, H11, H12, H61
	BI	4	445	MD: 4.16 [–0.26, 8.57]	74	H8, H11, H12, H61
Oral plus topical CHM as integrative medicine versus pharmacotherapy/rehabilitation	AS or MAS (upper limb)	4	329	SMD: –0.69 [–0.91, –0.47]*	0	H8, H9, H22, H40
	AS or MAS (lower limb)	5	449	SMD: –0.97 [–1.16, –0.77]*	0	H8, H9, H22, H38, H40
	AS or MAS (non-specified)	2	133	MD: –0.97 [–1.16, –0.77]*	0	H10, H61
	FMA (motor)	4	327	MD: 12.61 [8.84, 16.37]*	69	H6, H38, H55, H61
	BI	6	476	MD: 11.72 [8.37, 15.07]*	72	H6, H9, H38, H40, H55, H61

*Statistically significant.

Abbreviations: AS – Ashworth Scale; BI – Barthel Index; CHM – Chinese herbal medicine; CI – confidence interval; FMA – Fugl-Meyer Assessment; MAS – Modified Ashworth Scale; MD – mean difference; SMD – standardised mean difference.

Fugl-Meyer Assessment

Motor

Four studies (H8, H11, H12, H61) comparing oral plus topical CHM, to routine pharmacotherapy /rehabilitation reported the score of FMA (motor). The results showed that oral plus topical CHM was superior to routine pharmacotherapy and/or rehabilitation alone (MD: 4.20 [0.88, 7.52], I^2 = 38%) (Table 5.18). Four studies (H6, H38, H55, H61) that compared the combination of oral plus topical CHM and routine pharmacotherapy/rehabilitation to routine pharmacotherapy/ rehabilitation alone also reported FMA (motor function). It was found that the combination was more effective (MD: 12.61 [8.84, 16.37]), though with substantial heterogeneity (I^2 = 69%) (Table 5.18).

Upper limb

One study (H22) comparing the combination of oral plus topical CHM and rehabilitation, to rehabilitation alone, reported data on this outcome. The results showed that there was no significant difference between the combination and rehabilitation alone (MD: 8.77 [–6.20, 23.74]).

Lower limb

One study (H22) comparing the combination of oral plus topical CHM and routine pharmacotherapy and/or rehabilitation, to rehabilitation alone, reported data on this outcome. No significant difference between groups was found (MD: 10.02 [–3.95, 23.99]).

Barthel Index

Meta-analysis of four studies (H8, H11, H12, H61) did not detect significant differences between oral plus topical CHM and routine pharmacotherapy/rehabilitation (MD: 4.16 [–0.26, 8.57], but there was substantial heterogeneity (I^2 = 74%) (Table 5.18). The source of high heterogeneity could not be detected through sensitivity analysis.

Six studies (H6, H9, H38, H40, H55, H61) evaluated the add-on effects of oral plus topical CHM. Meta-analysis showed that adding oral CHM to routine pharmacotherapy/rehabilitation was more effective than routine pharmacotherapy/rehabilitation alone (MD: 11.72 [8.37, 15.07]), with substantial heterogeneity being detected (I^2 = 72%) (Table 5.18). The source of high heterogeneity could not be detected through sensitivity analysis.

Assessment Using Grading of Recommendations Assessment, Development and Evaluation

The overall certainty of clinical evidence of oral plus topical CHM, compared to routine pharmacotherapy, and oral plus topical CHM as integrative therapy for post-stroke spasticity is low (Tables 5.19 and 5.20).

Non-controlled Clinical Studies of Oral plus Topical Chinese Herbal Medicine

One case report (H69) was identified which assessed oral plus topical CHM for post-stroke spasticity. The study reported the effects of oral CHM (*Rou gan tong luo tang,* 柔肝通络汤) plus topical CHM (*Shu jin jie luan tang,* 舒筋解挛汤) on spasticity in the upper limbs and concluded that the oral and topical CHM treatment was effective for post-stroke spasticity. Ingredients of the oral formula: *Rou gan tong luo tang* 柔肝通络汤 were *zhi shou wu* 制首乌, *sang shen* 桑椹, *gou qi* 枸杞, *dan shen* 丹参, *ge gen* 葛根, *di long* 地龙, *chan tui* 蝉蜕, *xi xian cao* 豨莶草, *shen jin cao* 伸筋草, *bai shao* 白芍, *tian ma* 天麻, *shan zha* 山楂, *jiang can* 僵蚕, *ji nei jin* 鸡内金, *quan xie* 全蝎 and *fu ling* 茯苓, while those in the topical formula included *shen jin cao* 伸筋草, *hai tong pi* 海桐皮, *tou gu cao* 透骨草, *lu lu tong* 路路通, *xi xian cao* 豨莶草, *ai ye* 艾叶 and *bing pian* 冰片. However, the effects were not compared to any control method. Adverse events were not reported in this study.

Table 5.19 GRADE: Oral Plus Topical Chinese Herbal Medicine versus Routine Pharmacotherapy/Rehabilitation

Outcomes	No. of Participants (Studies)	Certainty of the Evidence (GRADE)	Anticipated Absolute Effects	
			Risk with Pharmacotherapy and/or Rehabilitation	Risk Difference with Oral plus Topical CHM (95% CI)
AS (upper limb)	120 (1 RCT)	⊕⊕○○ LOW[a,b]	The mean AS was **1.33.**	MD **0.20 lower** (0.57 lower to 0.17 higher)
AS (lower limb)	120 (1 RCT)	⊕⊕○○ LOW[a,b]	The mean AS was **103.**	MD **0.13 lower** (0.43 lower to 0.17 higher)
FMA (motor)	445 (4 RCTs)	⊕⊕⊕○ MODERATE[a]	The mean FMA was **70.20.**	MD **4.2 higher** (0.88 higher to 7.52 higher)
BI	445 (4 RCTs)	⊕⊕○○ LOW[a,c,d]	The mean BI was **60.49.**	MD **4.16 higher** (0.26 lower to 8.57 higher)

The risk in the intervention group (and its 95% confidence interval) is based on the assumed risk in the comparison group and the **relative effect** of the intervention (and its 95% CI).

Abbreviations: AS – Ashworth Scale; BI – Barthel Index; CHM – Chinese herbal medicine; CI – confidence interval; FMA – Fugl-Meyer Assessment; MD – mean difference; RCT – randomised controlled trial; SMD – standardised mean difference.

Notes
[a]Lack of blinding of participants, personnel and assessors.
[b]Small sample size limits certainty of results.
[c]High statistical heterogeneity.
[d]95% CI crosses no effect line.

Study References
AS (upper limb): H8
AS (lower limb): H8
FMA (motor): H8, H11, H12, H61
BI: H8, H11, H12, H61

Table 5.20 GRADE: Oral Plus Topical Chinese Herbal Medicine as Integrative Therapy versus Routine Pharmacotherapy/Rehabilitation

Outcomes	No. of Participants (Studies)	Certainty of the Evidence (GRADE)	Anticipated Absolute Effects: Risk with Pharmacotherapy and/or Rehabilitation	Anticipated Absolute Effects: Risk Difference with Oral plus Topical CHM as Integrative Therapy (95% CI)
AS or MAS (upper limb)	329 (4 RCTs)	⊕⊕○○ LOW[a,b]	–	SMD **0.69 lower** (0.91 lower to 0.47 lower)
AS or MAS (lower limb)	449 (5 RCTs)	⊕⊕⊕○ MODERATE[a]	–	SMD **0.97 lower** (1.16 lower to 0.77 lower)
FMA (motor)	327 (4 RCTs)	⊕⊕○○ LOW[a,c]	The mean FMA was **68.76.**	MD **12.61 higher** (8.84 higher to 16.37 higher)
FMA (upper limb)	60 (1 RCT)	⊕⊕○○ LOW[a,b]	The mean FMA was **27.49.**	MD **8.77 higher** (6.2 lower to 23.74 higher)
FMA (lower limb)	60 (1 RCT)	⊕⊕○○ LOW[a,b]	The mean FMA was **28.83.**	MD **10.02 higher** (3.95 lower to 23.99 higher)
BI	476 (6 RCTs)	⊕⊕○○ LOW[a,c]	The mean BI was **58.69.**	MD **11.72 higher** (8.37 higher to 15.07 higher)

The risk in the intervention group (and its 95% confidence interval) is based on the assumed risk in the comparison group and the **relative effect** of the intervention (and its 95% CI).

Abbreviations: AS – Ashworth Scale; BI – Barthel Index; CHM – Chinese herbal medicine; CI – confidence interval; FMA – Fugl-Meyer Assessment; MAS – Modified Ashworth Scale; MD – mean difference; RCT – randomised controlled trial; SMD – standardised mean difference.

Notes

[a]Lack of blinding of participants, personnel and assessors.

[b]Small sample size limits certainty of results.

[c]High statistical heterogeneity.

Study References

AS or MAS (upper limb): H8, H9, H22, H40

AS or MAS (lower limb): H8, H9, H22, H38, H40

FMA (motor): H6, H38, H55, H61

FMA (upper limb): H22

FMA (lower limb): H22

BI: H6, H9, H38, H40, H55, H61

Safety of Chinese Herbal Medicine

Among the 71 studies evaluating the efficacy of oral CHM, six studies (H1, H20, H31, H58, H59, H62) reported information on adverse events. There were two cases of mild nausea (H1) reported in patients taking oral CHM, but its association with oral CHM was not further explored. When CHM was used topically, one included study (H24) reported information on adverse events. There was one case presenting influenza-like symptoms during the treatment period reported in patients using topical CHM, but its association with topical CHM was not further explored.

Of the studies investigating oral plus topical CHM, six studies (H8–H11, H55, H61) reported information on adverse events. The others did not provide such information. Among those that applied oral and topical CHM, there were two cases of mild rash (one case in H9 and one case in H10); one case of worsening of spasticity (H10); two cases of dizziness and palpitation (H11); and one case of transient mild lowering of blood pressure (H61). However, details of these adverse events were not provided and their connection with oral or topical CHM was not further explored.

Overall, the use of CHM in post-stroke spasticity patients seems safe, but a lack of thorough and detailed reporting of adverse events prevents us from drawing a clear conclusion. Further clinical research should take this aspect into consideration and improve the quality of reporting on adverse events.

Evidence for Chinese Herbal Medicine Treatments Commonly Used in Clinical Practice

The common practice of CHM for stroke recommended by guidelines and textbooks was summarised in Chapter 2. Various topical CHM formulas were recommended by monographs[6,7] and one guideline.[8] In terms of oral CHM, various formulas were reported among the clinical studies, while published monographs[7] recommended only *Bu yang huan wu tang* 补阳还五汤 and *Di huang yin zi* 地黄饮子.

In this chapter, two studies (H5, H33) used the oral formula *Bu yang huan wu tang* 补阳还五汤, but none of them reported potential additional benefits in terms of AS or MAS. With regard to topical CHM, though different formulas were reported, most of the included studies did not provide names for their formulas. *Shu jin huo luo xi ji* 舒筋活络洗剂 was studied by two of the included trials (H23, H24) and demonstrated superior add-on effects in lower-limb MAS compared to routine care alone.

In terms of orally used herb ingredients, *bai shao* 白芍, as traditionally characterised by a function of relieving spasm and pain, was the most frequently used herb among clinical studies of oral CHM. This was followed by *dang gui* 当归, *gan cao* 甘草, *di long* 地龙 and *huang qi* 黄芪. As for topical herbs, *hong hua* 红花 was the most widely used ingredient in the included studies, followed by *dang gui* 当归, *mu gua* 木瓜, *shen jin cao* 伸筋草, *bai shao* 白芍 and *chuan xiong* 川芎. These herbs were consistent with those recommended by the monographs and guideline in Chapter 2.

Summary of Chinese Herbal Medicine Clinical Evidence

Evaluation of the clinical study evidence found variation in formulas and routes of administration of CHM, and diversity in outcomes reported. Both oral and topical CHM are frequently reported among the included studies. Treatment duration varied from two weeks to three months. Chinese medicine syndrome differentiation is not the highlight of clinical studies, since the majority of studies all selected similar treatment principles with Blood-moving and Collateral-activating herbs.

With regard to treatment effects, no superior effects could be detected with CHM, compared to traditional pharmacotherapy or placebo alone. However, adding oral or topical CHM, or a combination of oral and topical CHM, to traditional pharmacotherapy and/or rehabilitation therapy might receive additional benefits, compared to pharmacotherapy and/or rehabilitation therapy alone, in terms of spasticity severity of upper and lower extremities, motor function and activities of daily living.

For oral CHM formulas, only *Bu yang huan wu tang* 补阳还五汤 was repeatedly reported by multiple studies, which was also recommended by existing monographs and guidelines. In contrast, the topical CHM formula *Shu jin huo luo xi ji* 舒筋活络洗剂 for fumigation was not recommended by guidelines but reported by two of the included studies. However, there was not a particular formula confirmed as being the most effective, although all unnamed formulas have some herbs in common. Specifically, herbs used orally that may have contributed to the positive effects seen include *Bai shao* 白芍, *dang gui* 当归, *gan cao* 甘草, *di long* 地龙 and *huang qi* 黄芪. Some herbs are more often used topically, which may have contributed to the positive effects; these are *dang gui* 当归, *mu gua* 木瓜, *shen jin cao* 伸筋草, *bai shao* 白芍 and *chuan xiong* 川芎. It is worth noting that *bai shao* 白芍 and *dang gui* 当归 could be considered when preparing CHM prescriptions orally or topically for stroke patients with spasticity, based on the included studies of our research.

As for the safety of CHM therapy, mild adverse events including nausea, influenza-like symptoms, mild rash, dizziness, palpitation and worsening of spasticity were reported in studies using oral CHM, topical CHM, and the combination of oral and topical CHM. However, the connection of the above adverse events and CHM therapy was not explored and could not be confirmed. Future studies need to address the safety issues of CHM for post-stroke spasticity in more detail. Assessment using GRADE methods found that only the evidence with a combination of oral and topical CHM therapy for FMA (total motor function) was assessed as 'moderate certainty', others were assessed as 'low' or 'very low certainty'.

In summary, there is promising evidence supporting the use of CHM for the management of post-stroke spasticity. In clinical practice, the physician may consider incorporating therapies of oral and/or topical application of CHM with Blood-moving and Collateral-activating herbs, in addition to routine pharmacotherapy and rehabilitation for the management of post-stroke spasticity.

References

1. 陈紫薇, 谭子龙. (2016) 芍药甘草汤治疗中风后痉挛性偏瘫的系统评价. 云南中医中药杂志 **37(2):** 2.
2. Ashworth B. (1964) Preliminary trial of carisoprodal in multiple sclerosis. *Practitioner* **192:** 540–542.
3. Bohannon RW, Smith MB. (1987) Interrater reliability of a modified Ashworth scale of muscle spasticity. *Phys Ther* **67(2):** 206–207.
4. Sullivan KJ, Tilson JK, Cen SY, *et al.* (2011) Fugl-Meyer assessment of sensorimotor function after stroke: Standardized training procedure for clinical practice and clinical trials. *Stroke* **42(2):** 427–432.
5. Mahoney FI, Barthel DW. (1965) Functional evaluation: The Barthel index. *Md State Med J* **14:** 61–65.
6. 陈红霞, 中风病的中西医结合康复治疗. (2009) 北京: 人民卫生出版社.
7. 陈红霞, 神经系统疾病功能障碍中西医康复 (2016) 北京: 人民卫生出版社.
8. 中华中医药学会 中医内科常见病诊疗指南 — 西医疾病部分. (2008) 北京: 人民卫生出版社.

References for Included Chinese Herbal Medicine Clinical Studies

Study No.	References
H1	柳迎春. (2010) 加味黄芪桂枝五物汤治疗中风后痉挛性瘫痪 30 例临床观察. 江苏中医药 **(05):** 31–33.
H2	梁瑞琴. (2011) 安宫牛黄丸治疗脑血管意外的疗效观察. 实用心脑肺血管病杂志 **(09):** 1572–1573.
H3	王学新. (2013) 步长脑心通胶囊结合康复训练治疗脑卒中痉挛性偏瘫的疗效研究. 中国现代药物应用 **(13):** 36–37.
H4	马利中, 樊留博, 朱靖. (2009) 肌电生物反馈法或中药熏蒸法辅助治疗脑卒中偏瘫下肢痉挛的疗效比较. 中华物理医学与康复杂志 **31(2):** 2.
H5	陈恋戈. (2014) 加味补阳还五汤合康复训练治疗脑梗死痉挛期的临床观察. 按摩与康复医学 **5(5):** 2.
H6	支英豪. (2007) 解痉合剂对脑卒中肌痉挛病人运动功能和日常生活能力的影响. 中西医结合心脑血管病杂志 **15(9):** 2.
H7	张航. (2008) 解痉合剂结合康复疗法对脑卒中肌痉挛患者肌张力的影响. 浙江中医杂志 **(06):** 336.
H8	胡万华. (2009) 解痉合剂治疗脑卒中肌痉挛的临床研究. 中华中医药学刊 **(07):** 1403–1404.

(*Continued*)

(***Continued***)

Study No.	References
H9	朱文宗. (2007) 解痉合剂治疗脑卒中肌痉挛的随机对照临床研究. 中华中医药学刊 **(08):** 1648–1649.
H10	朱文宗, 胡万华, 周龙寿. (2002) 解痉合剂治疗脑卒中偏瘫后痉挛的临床研究. 中国康复理论与实践 **8(1):** 2.
H11	胡建芳. (2014) 解痉颗粒合中药熏蒸对中风后痉挛性瘫痪患者肢体功能的影响. 辽宁中医杂志 **(12):** 2629–2631.
H12	陈朝俊, 胡建芳, 刘媛. (2013) 解痉颗粒联合中药熏蒸对脑卒中痉挛性偏瘫肢体功能的影响. 中西医结合心脑血管病杂志 **(12):** 1420–1421.
H13	王成秀. (2013) 康复训练配合中药口服治疗脑卒中后肢体痉挛疗效观察. 中国中医急症 **(02):** 315–316.
H14	陈瑛玲, 陈立典, 陶静. (2013) 栝楼桂枝汤治疗中风后肢体痉挛的临床研究. 中医临床研究 **(04):** 7–9.
H15	斯琴高娃, 董秋梅. (2013) 蒙药忠伦阿汤熏蒸治疗脑卒中后上肢痉挛临床观察. 辽宁中医药大学学报 **(06):** 152–154.
H16	江云东. (2013) 祛风化瘀通络方早期干预急性缺血性脑卒中 42 例. 中国实验方剂学杂志 **(23):** 282–285.
H17	王海燕. (2008) 祛瘀生新煎治疗中风后肢体痉挛 46 例临床观察. 中医药通报 **(02):** 59–60.
H18	刘凤. (2015) 柔筋方湿热敷联合良肢位防治中风后痉挛性偏瘫的护理. 临床护理杂志 **(01):** 35–36.
H19	魏岳斌. (2011) 柔筋汤治疗脑卒中恢复期痉挛性偏瘫的临床研究. 中国中医药现代远程教育 **(07):** 17–18.
H20	张秋香. (2012) 芍药甘草汤合血府逐瘀汤加减治疗中风后痉挛性瘫痪 35 例临床观察. 河北中医 **(05):** 690–692.
H21	张颖, 杨坚, 高宁沁. (2012) 芍药甘草汤结合运动疗法治疗脑卒中后肘关节屈曲痉挛的临床研究. 上海中医药杂志 **(11):** 47–50.
H22	朱文宗. (2013) 芍药甘草汤结合运动训练治疗脑卒中后肌痉挛的临床疗效及表面肌电图分析. 中华物理医学与康复杂志 **35(6):** 4.
H23	欧海宁. (2007) 舒筋活络洗剂联合 A 型肉毒毒素注射对中风后踝跖屈肌痉挛的影响. 世界中医药 **(04):** 214–216.
H24	欧海宁. (2014) 舒筋活络洗剂联合 A 型肉毒毒素注射治疗脑卒中后上肢屈肌痉挛. 中国医药导报 **(20):** 98–102.

(*Continued*)

(**Continued**)

Study No.	References
H25	陈党红. (2009) 舒筋颗粒治疗卒中后肌张力增高 30 例临床观察. 山东中医药大学学报 **(04):** 300–301.
H26	黄健效. (2011) 舒筋通络方熏洗结合康复训练改善脑卒中后肢体痉挛临床研究. 中医学报 **(07):** 859–860.
H27	孙静. (2013) 四味宁舒散外敷治疗脑卒中后肌张力增高 30 例. 中医药通报 **(06):** 43–45, 54.
H28	李琰, 王松龄. (2011) 通络解痉汤结合康复训练治疗中风偏瘫痉挛 40 例. 中医研究 **(04):** 36–37.
H29	黄文. (2011) 温经舒筋胶囊治疗中风后偏瘫痉挛的疗效观察. 山东中医杂志 **(02):** 91–92.
H30	谭爱玲, 吕端, 养阴柔肝通络法治疗缺血性中风后痉挛 30 例临床观察. (2006) 江苏中医药**(08):** 24–25.
H31	乔文丽. (2014) 益气温阳 — 养阴解痉中药治疗中风偏瘫肢体痉挛随机平行对照研究. 实用中医内科杂志 **(12):** 12–14.
H32	张瑞杰. (2011) 中西医结合治疗中风后痉挛性偏瘫 50 例. 山东中医杂志 **(12):** 869–870.
H33	谭涛. (2012) 中药结合康复对脑卒中患者功能障碍及生活质量的影响. 中国中医药现代远程教育 **(05):** 12–13.
H34	刘斯尧. (2014) 中药结合康复训练治疗脑卒中后肢体痉挛疗效观察. 浙江中西医结合杂志 **(09):** 796–797.
H35	董其武. (2011) 中药结合康复训练治疗脑卒中肌痉挛 20 例疗效观察. 浙江中医杂志 **(07):** 508–509.
H36	冯利君, 易新华. (2007) 中药结合康复治疗对脑卒中患者的疗效. 中国康复 **(01):** 28.
H37	张颖, 乔蕾, 陈浩. (2008) 中药结合运动疗法治疗脑卒中上肢屈肌痉挛的疗效观察及表面肌电图分析. 中华物理医学与康复杂志 **30(6):** 4.
H38	谢仁明. (2011) 中药浸浴及内服结合康复训练治疗中风后肢体痉挛 60 例. 山东中医杂志 **(01):** 18–20.
H39	李华, 洪珍梅. (2014) 中药离子导入辅治中风痉挛性瘫痪. 浙江中西医结合杂志 **(01):** 68–69.
H40	杨标, 曲建平. (2006) 中药内服外用对脑卒中后痉挛性偏瘫的疗效观察. 辽宁中医杂志 **(11):** 1430.

(Continued)

(*Continued*)

Study No.	References
H41	李建英, 江群英, and 陈雯, 中药湿热敷配合被动运动对脑卒中后痉挛性瘫痪的疗效观察. (2002) 中国临床康复 **(11):** 1671.
H42	黄天国. (2011) 中药湿热敷治疗脑卒中后肢体痉挛的疗效分析. 求医问药(下半月) **(07):** 188.
H43	王林. (2014) 中药塌渍联合 Bobath 疗法治疗脑卒中后肌张力增高疗效观察. 按摩与康复医学 **5(10):** 3.
H44	沈金花, 王红敏, 朱凤磊. (2007) 中药外敷结合康复训练治疗中风痉挛状态的临床观察. 中国中西医结合杂志 **(09):** 834.
H45	范虹, 冯玲, 陶小英. (2013) 中药熏蒸及康复训练治疗卒中后上肢痉挛 23 例. 中国中医药科技 **(05):** 545–546.
H46	陈佳. (2010) 中药熏蒸结合巴氯芬治疗脑卒中偏瘫痉挛临床观察. 中国康复理论与实践 **(02):** 170–171.
H47	金力平. (2009) 中药熏蒸结合肌电生物反馈治疗中风后痉挛性偏瘫的临床分析. 浙江临床医学 **11(11):** 3.
H48	张颖, 高宁沁, 陈浩. (2007) 中药熏蒸结合运动疗法治疗脑卒中偏瘫痉挛临床研究. 上海中医药杂志 **(11):** 26–28.
H49	李翔, 钟格兰, 王利洪. (2008) 中药熏蒸治疗脑卒中偏瘫肌痉挛疗效分析. 中国误诊学杂志 **(31):** 7626–7627.
H50	高世毅, 何圣三. (2014) 中药熏蒸治疗卒中后痉挛性偏瘫 30 例临床观察. 河北中医 **(03):** 354–355.
H51	宋小娟, 寇丽霞. (2001) 中药药熨在脑梗塞早期康复护理中的应用. 现代护理 **(07):** 80–81.
H52	傅建明. (2014) 中药浴结合康复训练对脑卒中下肢痉挛患者步行能力的影响. 中国中医药科技 **(05):** 550–551.
H53	赵南. (2010) 中药足浴治疗脑卒中患者肢体痉挛的疗效观察. 中国中医药科技 **(06):** 504.
H54	贾爱明. (2012) 自拟解痉止痛方熏洗治疗脑卒中后肢体痉挛伴疼痛的临床观察. 疑难病杂志 **(05):** 346–348.
H55	张民旺. (2009) 中药治疗脑梗死(阴虚风动型)后痉挛性瘫痪的临床研究(Thesis). 河南中医学院, 第二临床医学院.
H56	杨晶. (2007) 中风龟羚熄风胶囊治疗中风后痉挛性瘫痪的临床研究(Thesis). 河南中医学院, 第一临床医学院.

(*Continued*)

(***Continued***)

Study No.	References
H57	金熙哲. (2005) 枳实芍药散结合康复训练治疗中风后偏瘫痉挛的研究 (Thesis). 北京中医药大学.
H58	盛芳. (2011) 养血通络汤治疗缺血中风后痉挛性瘫痪血虚络瘀证的临床观察 (Thesis). 湖南中医药大学.
H59	赵福臣. (2013) 温肾益气活血法治疗缺血性中风病痉挛性偏瘫的临床研究 (Thesis). 山东中医药大学.
H60	陈瑛玲. (2013) 栝楼桂枝汤治疗脑卒中后下肢痉挛的临床研究 (Thesis). 福建中医药大学.
H61	翁贤君. (2014) 解痉合剂联合盐酸替扎尼定片治疗中风后痉挛性偏瘫（阴虚风动型）的疗效评价 (Thesis). 浙江中医药大学.
H62	姜美玲. (2014) 大秦艽汤加减对卒中上肢痉挛性瘫痪患者运动功能的影响 (Thesis). 广州中医药大学.
H63	张兰坤, 过伟峰, 盛蕾. (2013) 从肝肾阴虚、风痰瘀阻论治卒中后痉挛性瘫痪. 中国中医药信息杂志 **(1):** 94–95.
H64	孙西庆. (2011) 从阳虚风痰阻络探讨中风病肢体痉挛的发病机理. 中国中医急诊 **(8):** 1354–15.
H65	李彦萍. (2009) 化瘀通脉汤加减在治疗卒中后肢体痉挛的临床应用. 中国医药指南 **(15):** 124–125.
H66	宋国平, 赵晓兴, 程新元. (1998) 破血逐瘀法治疗脑梗塞后肢体痉挛的临床观察. 北京中医药大学学报 **(5):** 60.
H67	宋国平, 刘志宏. (1996) 破血逐瘀法治愈偏瘫痉挛 1 例. 北京中医药大学学报 **(5):** 51.
H68	崔昕. (1996) 芍药甘草汤提取剂对脑血管障碍引起的腓肠肌痉挛的疗效. 国外医学中医中药分册 **(2):** 20.
H69	李振华. (2013) 周慎治疗中风后手痉挛经验. 辽宁中医药杂志 **(1):** 34–35.
H70	王颖, 张闻东, 陈幸生. (2005) 自拟益气养阴方治疗中风后肢体痉挛初步观察. 中医药临床杂志 **(1):** 18–19.
H71	于曼. (2014) 中药拘挛方泡洗缓解中风急性期后踝关节拘挛症状临床观察 (Thesis). 北京中医药大学.

6

Pharmacological Actions of the Common Herbs

OVERVIEW

The great therapeutic effects of Chinese herbal formulas and herbs for post-stroke spasticity are largely attributed to their active compounds. This section reviews the available experimental evidence to explore the possible biological activities and mechanisms of the ten most frequently used Chinese herbs from the randomised clinical trials in Chapter 5.

Introduction

This chapter reviews experimental evidence from *in vitro* cell and *in vivo* animal models for the ten most frequently used herbs identified in Chapter 5, including *bai shao* 白芍, *dang gui* 当归, *mu gua* 木瓜, *gan cao* 甘草, *hong hua* 红花, *shen jin cao* 伸筋草, *di long* 地龙, *chuan xiong* 川芎, *huang qi* 黄芪 and *dan shen* 丹参, to possibly explain the findings from the randomised controlled clinical trials (RCTs) for post-stroke spasticity.

The extracts or/and isolated compounds from each herb have shown vast pharmacological effects, in particular, compounds with anti-inflammatory and antioxidant effects, and potential cardioprotective activities including anti-atherogenesis, anti-hyperlipidemic, anti-thrombosis, anti-hypertension and anti-myocardial ischaemia. They are generally beneficial to the whole body for stroke prevention and recovery by improving cardiovascular and cerebrovascular homeostasis. In relation to the pathological processes and mechanisms of post-stroke spasticity described in Chapter 1, neuron motor impairments (central region) and muscle spasticity and weakness (periphery region) are the main issues. In order to identify experimental studies for their pharmacological actions of relevance to post-stroke spasticity, the pharmacological activities of each herb or compound will be presented with regard to their therapeutic effects for promoting neuromotor recovery and relieving muscle tension and/or improving muscle strength if available.

Searches were conducted of PubMed to identify studies. Search terms included the names of the plant in Chinese *pinyin* and scientific names, and the names of compounds contained in the plant. These were combined with terms for neuroprotection, spasmodic activity and analgesic activity.

Experimental Studies on *Bai Shao* 白芍

Bai shao 白芍 (white peony) is mainly derived from the dried root without bark of *P. lactiflora* Pall. The main characteristic constituents of *P. lactiflora* Pall contain monoterpenoids, triterpenoids, flavonoids, phenols and tannins. It consists of more than 15 components, with the main bioavailable compounds being paeoniflorin, pentagalloylglucose, gallic acid, albiflorin and benzoic acid. Most of the compounds are monoterpene glucosides, and among them, paeoniflorin, a chief active ingredient in the root of *P. lactiflora* Pall, which is the most abundant (> 90%) in accounting for the pharmacological activities (see reviews[1,2]). These compounds have been extensively studied and show multiple functions with greater potential anti-inflammatory, antioxidant, antiviral, antibacterial, antifungal, anti-tumor, anti-arthritis, anti-coagulant, anti-platelet and immunomodulatory activity (see reviews[1,2]). Other pharmacological effects in relation to post-stroke spasticity are reviewed below.

Neuroprotective Activity

In rat primary cultures, two monoterpenes, paeonilactone-C and benzoylpaeoniflorin, significantly protected cortical cells against hydrogen peroxide (H_2O_2)-induced neurotoxicity.[3] In cultured primary hippocampal neurons, paeoniflorin (100–200 μM) protected cells from N-methyl-d-aspartic acid (NMDA)-induced excitotoxicity via the modulation of the Ca^{2+}/CaMKI)/cAMP response element-binding protein (CREB) signalling pathway.[4]

In both transient and permanent middle cerebral artery occlusion (MCAO)-induced focal cerebral ischaemia-reperfusion (I/R) injury rat models, the administration of paeoniflorin (2.5 and 5 mg/kg) produced a dose-dependent decrease in both neurological impairment and the histologically measured infarction volume by activating adenosine A1 receptors.[5] With a similar animal model, the same group found that pre-treatment with paeonol (20 mg/kg) and paeoniflorin (10 mg/kg) decreased infarction volume and neurological deficit scores by scavenging superoxide anions, inhibiting microglial activation and decreasing interleukin-1beta (IL-1β), nuclear factor-kappa B (NFκB) and tumor necrosis factor-alpha (TNF-α) expressions.[6] A more recent study using the MCAO-I/R model further proved the distinguished neuroprotective effect of paeoniflorin (5 mg/kg) which attenuated cerebral ischaemia-induced neuronal apoptosis by regulating the Ca^{2+}/CaMKI)/CREB signalling pathway which was closely related to anti-apoptotic signalling.[4]

Anti-spasmodic Activity

It is reported that *P. lactiflora* can effectively relieve muscle cramps of various types, particularly when combined with licorice (*gan cao* 甘草). Paeoniflorin and glycyrrhizin (a major active glycoside in licorice) individually, were too low to inhibit muscle contraction but were very active when applied simultaneously on isolated sciatic nerve-sartorius muscle preparations in frogs, or on isolated or *in situ* phrenic nerve-diaphragm muscle preparations in mice.[7] Recently, a direct study in a post-stroke hypermytonia animal model, which had obvious hemiplegia with spasm in rats after cerebral I/R, demonstrated that licorice alone and combined with *P. lactiflora* improved the scores of postural reflex assessment in rats, while the muscle tension and mobility of rats were significantly improved after nine days' treatment with *P. lactiflora* combined with licorice, comparable to baclofen. The improvement was accompanied with a decrease in the content of excitatory amino acids (glutamic acid and aspartic acid) in serum and glycine in brain tissues of rats.[8]

Analgesic Activity

It has been shown that the analgesic effect of paeoniflorin (180 mg/kg) in rats with neonatal maternal separation-induced visceral hyperalgesia was mediated, at least in part, through adenosine A1 receptors by inhibiting the extracellular signal-regulated protein kinase (ERK) pathway.[9]

Experimental Studies on *Dang Gui* 当归

Dang gui 当归, mainly derived from the dried root of *Angelica sinensis (Radix Angelica sinensis),* consists of over 70 compounds. Ferulic acid, *Z*-Ligustilide, butylidenephthalide, butyl-phthalide and polysaccharide are thought to be the main biologically active components in *Angelica sinensis,* and ferulic acid has been used as the marker compound for the quality control (see reviews[10–12]). These compounds have diverse biological activities including anti-inflammatory, antioxidant, anti-arthrosclerosis, anti-thrombotic, anti-platelet, anti-hepatotoxic, anti-cardiovascular and immunomodulatory activity (see reviews[10–12]). Other pharmacological effects in relation to post-stroke spasticity are reviewed below.

Neuroprotective Activity

Z-ligustilide (Z-LIG) exerted a pronounced neuroprotective effect on H_2O_2-induced injury in PC12 cells. Pre-treatment of the cells with Z-LIG (0.1, 1.0, 2.5 or 5.0 μg/ml) significantly protected cells against H_2O_2-induced cytotoxicity via improving cellular antioxidant defence and inhibiting the mitochondrial apoptotic pathway.[13]

Dang gui 当归 has been demonstrated to be protective in the ischaemic brain against transient and permanent MCAO-induced focal cerebral I/R injury in rats and ICR mice, possibly through antioxidant and anti-apoptotic mechanisms *in vivo.*

Ferulic acid (FA) (80 and 100 mg/kg) reduced the size of cerebral infarct and neurological deficit score through inhibiting superoxide radicals, intercellular adhesion molecule-1 (ICAM-1) and NF-κB in transient MCAO in rats.[14] Z-ligustilide (20 or 80 mg/kg) at two hours after ischaemia in rats reduced cerebral infarct volumes and brain swelling, and improved behavioural deficits.[15] Five and 20 mg/kg of Z-LIG treatment could protect I/R-induced brain injury by increasing the activities of the antioxidant enzyme glutathione peroxidase (GSH-PX) and superoxide dismutase (SOD), and apoptosis by decreasing Bax and caspase-3 in brain tissues of mice.[16] The researcher further investigated the effect of Z-LIG on chronic cerebral hypoperfusion with post-ischaemic administration of Z-LIG (10 and 40 mg/kg) in Wistar rats. Z-LIG was shown to increase the choline acetyltransferase activity and inhibit the acetyl-choline esterase activity in ischaemic brain tissue.[17]

In addition to neuroprotective effects, Z-ligustilide could promote adult neurogenesis in the hippocampus following chronic cerebral hypoperfusion in MCAO rats. The effects of neurogenic enhancement might be due to increased brain-derived neurotrophic factor (BDNF) and phosphorylated CREB levels.[18] Furthermore, sodium ferulate (SF, sodium salt of FA) and butylidenephthalide also demonstrated an ability to enhance neurogenesis when combined with bone marrow stromal cell (BMSC) after seven days of ischaemic stroke in MCAO models.[19]

Anti-spasmodic Activity

Ligustilide, butylidenephthalide and butylphthalide were found to be capable of relaxing rat uterine contractions and other smooth muscle systems as non-specific anti-spasmodics.[20]

Analgesic Activity

A water extract of *Angelica sinensis* containing 81% polysaccharide possessed significant analgesic activity by decreasing the frequency of the wringing reaction induced by acetic acid and increasing the pain threshold in the hot-plate procedure in mice.[21]

Experimental Studies on *Mu Gua* 木瓜

Chaenomeles is the effective medicinal source for *mu gua* 木瓜 used in China to treat various diseases. The main chemical constituents isolated from *Chaenomeles* consist of flavonoids, triterpenoids, phenolic and phenylpropionic acids, saccharides, essential oils and alkaloids. Among them, oleanolic and ursolic acids belonging to the triterpenoid acid family are the characteristic chemical markers used for the quality of *Chaenomeles* (see reviews[22,23]). Oleanolic acid (OA) and ursolic acid (UA) are also the major active constituents which have shown multiple functions with great potential regarding anti-inflammatory, antioxidant, antimicrobial, anti-influenza, anti-Parkinsonian, anti-tumour, anti-nociceptive, hepatoprotective and immunoregulatory properties (see reviews[22,23]). Other pharmacological effects in relation to post-stroke spasticity are reviewed below.

Neuroprotective Activity

Oleanolic acid, a triterpenoid compound, has shown neuroprotective effects *in vitro* and *in vivo*. In H_2O_2-injured PC12 cells, pre-treatment with OA (1 and 10 μM) significantly protects cells from H_2O_2-induced injury. In the cerebral ischaemia mouse model by bilateral common carotid arteries ligation (BCCAL) and MCAO rats, pre-administration with OA (25, 50 mg/kg) in BCCAL mice significantly prolonged animal survival time in mice, and OA (12.5 and 25 mg/kg) in MCAO rats remarkably reduced infarct area, cerebral oedema and cerebral ischaemic damage, and improved neurological function, which may be in part through modulating endogenous antioxidants and improving mitochondrial function.[24] In addition to the neuroprotective effect, OA (10 nM) promotes differentiation of neural stem cells (NSC) from mouse embryos at embryonic day 14 (E14) towards neurons partially through Nkx-2.5-dependent mechanism.[25] Furthermore, UA, another triterpenoid compound, has been proven to protect the brain against ischaemic injury in transient MCAO wild-type mice with improved neurological function and reduced the size of the infarct by activating the nuclear factor-erythroid 2-related factor 2 (Nrf2) pathway and decreasing the expression of Toll-like receptor 4 (TLR4) and NF-κB.[26]

Anti-spasmodic Activity

The active fraction from *Chaenomeles* is a potential agonist of human β2-adrenoceptors, which is involved in smooth muscle relaxation with an EC_{50} of 4.8 μg/ml.[27] Flavonoids, another main bioactive constituent of *Chaenomeles*, have shown inhibitory effects on gastrointestinal smooth muscle contraction in isolated rabbit gastric fundus and ileum, induced by acetylcholine and $CaCl_2$, in a dose-dependent manner, and in the isolated rabbit taenia coli elicited by high K^+ depolarisation. These relaxant effects may be associated with the voltage-dependent Ca^{2+} channel blockade by total flavonoids.[28,29]

Analgesic Activity

Glucosides isolated from *Chaenomeles* at 60, 120 and 240 mg/kg for mice and 30, 60 and 120 mg/kg for rats inhibit acetic acid-induced writhing responses and second phase of formalin-induced responses in mice, and suppress the increased arthritic flexion scores in rats. This is likely associated with their inhibitory effects on peripheral inflammatory mediators.[30] Similar fractions of extract of *Chaenomeles* showed remarkable analgesic activity in the acetic acid-induced abdominal contraction test and formalin-induced paw licking test in mice and rats.[31]

Experimental studies on *Gan Cao* 甘草

The three original plants of *gan cao* 甘草 (licorice) in Chinese medicine are *Glycyrrhiza uralensis* Fisch., *Glycyrrhiza inflata* Bat. and *Glycyrrhiza glabra* L. Among the at least 400 isolated compounds, the main bioactive constituents of licorice are triterpene saponins (more than 20) and various types of flavonoids (more than 300) (see reviews[32–34]). These compounds exhibit extensive pharmacological properties such as anti-inflammatory, anti-allergic, antioxidative, antiviral, anti-carcinogenic, anti-thrombotic, anti-ulceric, immunoregulatory, hepatoprotective and cardioprotective effects (see reviews[32,34,35]). Other pharmacological effects in relation to post-stroke spasticity are reviewed below.

Neuroprotective Activity

The neuroprotective activity of licorice has been largely attributed to an active component of *gan cao* flavonoids: isoliquiritigenin (ISL). It has been shown that ISL (10 μM) protects HT22 hippocampal neuronal cells from glutamate-induced mitochondrial damage and cell death caused by glutamate via inhibiting the expression of the apoptotic regulators Bcl-2 and Bax and suppressing glutamate-induced reactive oxygen species (ROS) production.[36] It also protects cultured cortical neurons from Aβ (25–35)-induced neuronal apoptotic death by interfering with the increases of ($[Ca^{2+}]_i$) and ROS,[37] indicating ISL's protection of neuron damage *in vitro*.

In addition, two neuroprotective compounds have been demonstrated to be effective in rat models of cerebral ischaemia. In transient MCAO-induced focal cerebral I/R injury, pre-treatment with ISL (5, 10 and 20 mg/kg) significantly reduced the cerebral infarct volume and oedema, and produced significant reduction in neurological deficits due to the amelioration of cerebral energy metabolism and its antioxidant property.[38] Another compound, liquiritin (10, 20 and 40 mg/kg), from flavonoids showed a similar neuroprotective effect. In MCAO-I/R mice, liquiritin administered before MCAO once a day for three days decreased neurological deficits and infarct volume due to its antioxidant and anti-apoptotic properties.[39]

Anti-spasmodic Activity

Several anti-spasmodic activities have been attributed to the combination of licorice and *P. lactiflora* to improve muscle tension and mobility in post-stroke hypermytonia animal models (refer to *bai shao* 白芍).

Experimental Studies on *Hong Hua* 红花

Hong hua 红花 (*Carthamus tinctorius* L.; safflower) contains many chemical constituents including quinochalcones, flavonoids, alkaloids, polyacetylenes, alkanediol, fatty acids, steroids and lignans. Among them, quinochalcones and flavonoids are considered as the characteristic and active constituents with the quinochalcone C-glycoside hydroxysafflor yellow A (HSYA), N-(p-Coumaroyl) serotonin and N-feruloylserotonin responsible for most of the pharmacological activities of *C. tinctorius* (see reviews[40,41]).

With the current information, it is evident that extracts and compounds of *C. tinctorius* seeds and flowers have great pharmacological importance for cardiovascular protection, cerebrovascular protection, hepatoprotection, anti-tumour, anti-osteoporosis, anti-diabetes, antimicrobial, anti-coagulant, antioxidant and anti-atherosclerosis effects (see reviews[40,41]). Other pharmacological effects in relation to post-stroke spasticity are reviewed below.

Neuroprotective Activity

The major component of the yellow pigment HSYA has attracted the most attention and has proved to be a promising therapeutic agent for cerebrovascular diseases. In the cultured primary rat cortical neuronal, HSYA (10 μM) showed protective effects for cortical neurons via inhibiting the expression of NR2B-containing NMDA receptors by regulating the Bcl-2 family.[42] As for PC12 cells, HSYA (20, 40 and 80 μM) significantly protected cells from neurotoxicity induced by β-amyloid as evidenced by reversed changes triggered by β-amyloid.[43]

The protective effect of HSYA against cerebral I/R injury in an MCAO model has indicated that HSYA suppressed thrombosis formation in MCAO rats, beginning with a dose of 3 mg/kg. It also improved the neurological deficit scores and reduced the cerebral infarct area in a dose-dependent manner by inhibition of platelet aggregation and regulation of PGI2/TXA2 ratio.[44] Furthermore, other studies reported the protective effect of HSYA (4 and 8 mg/kg) occurred partly through reducing apoptosis via the PI3K/Akt/GSK3b signalling pathway[45] and decreased nitrotyrosine formation.[46] A recent study with extracts suggested this neuroprotective effect occurred through antioxidative and anti-inflammatory mechanisms.[47]

In addition to HSYA, N-(p-Coumaroyl) serotonin and N-feruroylserotonin have been reported to possess neuroprotective activity. Post-ischaemic treatment with kaempferol-3-O-rutinoside (KRS, 10.0 mg/kg) and kaempferol-3-O-glucoside (KGS, 7.5 mg/kg) reduced neurological deficits and brain infarct volume, and protected neuron and axon damage after ischaemia-reperfusion in MACO rats by inhibition of signal transducer and activator of transcription (STAT)3 and NF-kB activation.[48]

Analgesic Activity

Carthamus tinctorius L. possesses central analgesic activity. Safflow yellow A (50–100 mg/kg) demonstrated sustained analgesic actions in mice.[49] In another study it was also found that 50–100 mg/kg dose of *C. tinctorius* flower sustained analgesic activity with a remarkable reduction in nociceptive and proprioceptive activity. This occurred through proteolytic degradation of tyrosinase, which is responsible for the inhibition of monoaminergic neurotransmitters (pain signal transmitters).[50]

Experimental Studies on *Shen Jin Cao* 伸筋草

Shen jin cao 伸筋草 (*Lycopodium japonicum* Thunb.), used as a traditional Chinese medicine for the treatment of contusion, strains and myasthenia, is a rich source of lycopodium alkaloids.[51] Lycopodium alkaloids have attracted many groups' attention to synthesise it due to its highly diverse and unique skeletal characteristics. Alkaloids, such as lycojaponicumins A–E, lycopodine-type alkaloids, fawcettimine-related alkaloids and a number of others, have been isolated and identified from *Lycopodium japonicum* Thunb.[52–55] However, the number of available studies on the pharmacological activities is limited and further investigations are required.

Lycopdine from the extracts of alkaloids has shown to inhibit acetylcholinesterase (AChE), a neurotransmitter disrupted after stroke.[55–57] Furthermore, studies with the extract in mice also demonstrated inhibitory effects on AChE activity in the cortex, striatum and hippocampus, as well as decreased lipid peroxidation in these locations and in the cerebellum.[58]

Experimental Studies on *Di Long* 地龙

Di long 地龙 (*Pheretima*) consists of *P. aspergillum*, *P. vulgaris* (Chen), *P. guillelmi* (Michaelsen) and *P. pectinifera* (Michaelsen). *P. aspergillum* is considered to be the best source of *Pheretima* and is used in traditional oriental medicine for the treatment of a variety of diseases including asthma, cough, stroke and seizure (see reviews[59,60]). The bioactive chemical constituents of *P. aspergillum* have not been comprehensively investigated due to its complex components, although it has been reported to contain lumbrofebrin, lumbritin, hypoxanthine and also several peptides. The extract of *P. aspergillum* has various beneficial pharmacological activities, including fibrinolytic, anti-coagulative, hepatoprotective, antioxidative and anti-inflammatory activities, as well as wound healing and peripheral nerve regeneration abilities (see reviews[59,60]). Other pharmacological effects in relation to post-stroke spasticity are reviewed below.

Neuroprotective Activity

It has been shown that *P. aspergillum* extract could promote the differentiation of neurite-bearing cells and the proliferation and migration ability of RSC96 Schwann cells.[61–63] *P. aspergillum* extract could enhance nerve growth factor-mediated neurite outgrowth in PC12 cells and promote regeneration of dissected rat sciatic nerve in silicone rubber chambers, indicating *P. aspergillum* plays a major role in nerve regeneration.[63]

Additionally, in MCAO rats, oral administration of *P. aspergillum* at 0.25, 0.5 and 1 g/kg could protect against MCAO-induced cerebral infarction with a decrease in neuronal death, glial proliferation and S100B proteins in the ischaemic core in the cortex.[64] Furthermore, lumbrokinase, a group of potential fibrinolytic enzymes derived from *Pheretima*, has demonstrated anti-ischaemic activity by protecting the brain and vessels against ischaemic injury in MCAO rats. This occurs by inhibiting platelet aggregation and facilitating platelet disaggregating through increasing platelet cAMP levels and activity of adenylate cyclase.[65]

In addition to the neuroprotective effect, *P. aspergillum* extracts at 125 μg/ml can stimulate RSC96 Schwann cell migration and regeneration by inducing the expression of matrix-degrading proteolytic enzymes, and metalloproteinase (MMP) 2 and MMP 9 through extracellular signal regular protein (ERK1/2) and p38 of the MAPK signalling pathway.[62] The main mechanism of *P. aspergillum* in enhancing Schwann regeneration is dependent on the P13K protein.[61] Lumbricusin, a *Pheretima* peptide, has been reported to enhance neuronal proliferation of human neuroblastoma SH-SY5Y cells[66] and mouse NSCs[67] by increasing ubiquitination of $p27^{Kip1}$ protein, a negative regulator of cell-cycle progression, and by ameliorating neuroinflammation through inhibition of microglial activation.[68]

Experimental Studies on *Chuan Xiong* 川芎

Ligusticum chuanxiong Hort (LC; Umbelliferae) sourced for *chuan xiong* 川芎 is an effective medical plant. More than 200 compounds have been isolated and identified from LC and can be grouped into five basic types: phenols and organic acids, phthalides, alkaloids, polysaccharides, ceramides and cerebrosides. Ferulic acid, ligustilide and tetramethylpyrazine (TMP, also known as ligustrazine) are the main active constituents of LC, especially in the treatment of neurovascular and cardiovascular diseases (see reviews[69,70]). These compounds demonstrate a broad therapeutic capacity, including effects on cardiovascular and cerebrovascular diseases, vasodilatation, thrombus formation, myocardial I/R injury, antioxidation, anti-inflammation, anti-bacterial, anti-fibrotic, anti-neoplastic, anti-pyretic and anti-diabetic activity, and also angiogenic, chondroprotective and progesterone-like activity (see reviews[69,70]). Other pharmacological effects in relation to post-stroke spasticity are reviewed below.

Neuroprotective Activity

Ferulic acid, ligustilide and TMP have attracted significant research attention in terms of minimising stroke damage. Ferulic acid (80 and 100 mg/kg) has been reported to reduce the size of cerebral infarct and neurological deficit score through inhibiting superoxide radicals, ICAM-1 and NF-κB in transient MCAO animal models.[14]

Ligustilide (20, 40 or 80 mg/kg) demonstrated a protective effect against the damage induced by I/R to the rat brain *in vivo* and rat cultured neurons *in vitro* by promoting erythropoietin transcription via an ERK signalling pathway. It also inhibited the expression of the stress-induced protein RTP801,[71] and increased the activity of the antioxidant enzyme GSH-PX and SOD, and apoptosis by decreasing Bax and caspase-3 in the mouse ICR ischaemic brain as well.[16]

The protective effects of TMP against neural damage have been extensively studied in recent years with multiple mechanisms. Using a glioma–neuronal co-culturing system, TMP (100 μM) has shown to effectively inhibit glioma cells and protect primary cultured cerebral neurocytes against H_2O_2-induced damage by downregulating chemokine receptor CXCR4 expression.[72] Other studies demonstrated TMP (25 and 50 μM) neuroprotection against kainate-induced excitotoxicity by stabilising mitochondrial function with quenching of ROS and reducing intracellular calcium, and inhibiting glutamate-induced neuronal death *in vivo* and *in vitro*.[73] Additionally, activation of Nrf2/HO-1 expression[74] and preservation of postsynaptic protein synthesis by reversing the cAMP/PKA/CREB pathway remarkably contributed to TMP-mediated neuroprotection against cerebral ischaemia (20 mg/kg) or scopolamine-induced neuronal injuries.[75] In addition to the neuroprotective effects, TMP could also stimulate cell differentiation and enhance neurogenesis in MCAO rats.[76] It could induce NSC differentiation towards neurons in hypoxic conditions by regulating the phosphorylation of ERK and p38,[77] and promote human neuroblastoma SH-SY5Y cell differentiation into neurons through epigenetic regulation of Topoisomerase Iiβ.[78]

Anti-spasmodic Activity

There are very few studies dealing with the influence of *chuan xiong* 川芎 on muscle relaxation. Ligustilide has been reported to have centrally acting muscle relaxant effects on the crossed extensor reflex in anesthetised rats.[79]

Analgesic Activity

Tetramethylpyrazin shows anti-nociceptive effects with elevation of the threshold of thermal nociception by inhibiting high-voltage gated calcium currents and tetrodotoxin-resistant sodium currents of dorsal root ganglion neurons in rats.[80]

Experimental Studies on *Huang Qi* 黄芪

Astragali radix (AR), known as *huang qi* 黄芪 in China, is sourced from the dried root of *Astragalus membranaceus* and *Astragalus membranaceus var. mongholicus*. More than 200 compounds have been isolated and identified from AR with the significant bioactive constituents being saponins, flavonoids, polysaccharides and amino acids. Among them, the triterpenoid saponin astragaloside IV is a principal active component of the herb and is known to be the qualitative control biomarker (see reviews[81,82]). In pharmacological studies crude extracts of AR, as well as isolated constituents, have multiple pharmacological effects including anti-inflammatory, anti-oxidative, anti-fibrotic, anti-asthma, anti-cancer, anti-diabetic, anti-hyperglycemic, anti-aging, anti-tumor and antiviral activities, and immunostimulant, cardioprotective and hepatoprotective effects (see reviews[81,83]). Other pharmacological effects in relation to post-stroke spasticity are reviewed below.

Neuroprotective Activity

Astragaloside IV (AST-IV) shows the most therapeutic potential for stroke with a growing body of divergent pre-clinical evidence indicating it has neuroprotective and cardioprotective activities, amongst others (see reviews[83,84]). A very recent review article summarised the effect of AST-IV on cerebral ischaemia animals. In 13 studies with 244 animals (rats and mice), AST-IV exerted potential neuroprotection by improving neurological deficits and infarct volume, and reduced blood-brain barrier permeability in experimental focal cerebral MCAO-I/R animals. This was largely mediated by multiple mechanisms, such as antioxidative/nitration stress reaction, and anti-inflammatory and anti-apoptotic activities (see the details in the review[84]).

In addition to AST-IV, calycosin, a major isoflavonoid in AR, also has significant experimental evidence indicating therapeutic potential for stroke based on its neuroprotective activity.[85] In a transient rat MCAO model, calycosin (30 mg/kg) induced neuroprotection by attenuating the neurological deficit and infarct volume, whilst reducing malondialdehyde (MDA) and ROS, and upregulating catalase, SOD and GSH-Px activity in a dose-dependent manner.[86] Further studies from the same group on MCAO rats and *in vitro* primary cultured neurons demonstrated that calycosin's protection of the brain from I/R injury occurred through the transient receptor potential canonical 6 (TRPC6)-CREB pathway by increasing TRPC6 and P-CREB expression and inhibiting calpain activation.[87]

Anti-spasmodic Activity

Relaxant effects of calycosin on isolated rat thoracic aorta rings pre-contracted with phenylephrine (PHE) or KCl have indicated that calycosin is a non-competitive Ca(2+) channel blocker which might relieve muscle cramps after stroke.[88] Kaempferol, another isoflavonoid in AR, also has relaxant effects on KCl (60 mM)-induced tonic contraction in isolated rat uterus in a concentration-dependent manner by modulating cAMP, transcription and protein synthesis.[89]

Experimental Studies on *Dan Shen* 丹参

Dan shen 丹参 (*Salvia*) consists of several species including *S. miltiorrhiza, S. leriifolia, S. officinalis, S. haematodes, S. triloba* and *S. divinorum. S. miltiorrhiza* has been extensively used in traditional oriental medicine for the treatment of a variety of diseases. The dried roots and flowers of *S. miltiorrhiza* contain diverse chemical components including 49 diterpenoid quinones from the roots, 36 hydrophilic phenolic acids from the roots and 23 essential oil constituents from the flowers. Based on their structural characteristics, the principal bioactive constituents can be classified into two groups. The first group contains lipid-soluble lipophilic constituents (known as tanshinones) such as tanshinone I, tanshinone IIA, tanshinone IIB, cryptotanshinone and dihydrotanshinone. The second group contains water-soluble polyphenolic constituents (known as salvianolic acids/depsides) such as salvianolic acid B (Sal B), Sal A and *dan shen su* (see reviews[90–92]). *S. miltiorrhiza* extracts and its constituents have been extensively studied and show multiple important pharmacological effects on anti-inflammatory, antioxidant, anti-Alzheimer's disease, anti-Parkinson's disease, anti-neuropathic pain, anti-diabetes mellitus, anti-cancer, anti-fibrotic and anti-hepatocyte activities, as well as acute lung and renal injury, and anti-alcohol dependence. In addition to these general pharmacological effects, its potential cardioprotective activities, including anti-atherogenesis, anti-hyperlipidemic, anti-thrombosis, anti-hypertension and anti-myocardial ischaemic injury, may improve cardiovascular homeostasis and reduce stroke risk (see reviews[90,93]). Other pharmacological effects in relation to post-stroke spasticity are reviewed below.

Neuroprotective Activity

With a large amount of experimental evidence in several different animal models, particularly using MCAO, *S. miltiorrhiza* extract and its compounds have shown multiple neuroprotective potentials. Two groups of bioactive constituents of *S. miltiorrhiza* contribute to the neuroprotective activities (see review[93]). Studies on MCAO rats, amyloid precursor protein (APP) transgenic mice and Mongolian gerbils show that these constituents could improve cognitive impairment, reduce neurological deficits and exert their neuroprotective effects by crossing the blood-brain barrier. Due to their different structures, sizes and polarity, the biochemical mechanisms involved in the neuroprotective activity are different and complementary, but mainly occur through anti-inflammatory, antioxidant, anti-apoptotic and angiogenetic mechanisms (as summarised in the review[93]).

In addition to the extensive studies reporting on the neuroprotective effects of *S. miltiorrhiza,* a number of studies have reported the neurogenic activities of *S. miltiorrhiza* which would be beneficial to recovery of neurons affected by stroke. Recent research has indicated that Sal B regulates proliferation of rat embryonic cortex neural stem/progenitor cells (NSPCs) in a dose- and time-dependent manner by activating the PI3K/Akt signalling pathway *in vitro,* and could maintain the proliferation of NSPCs and improve cognitive impairment after cerebral ischaemia in rats.[94] Further studies on Sal B also show that it could promote the proliferation and neural differentiation of transplanted exogenous bone marrow-derived neural stem cells (BM-NSCs) by inducing BDNF production.[95] Moreover, extracts of *S. miltiorrhiza* (5 μg/ml) could enhance the differentiation of mouse-induced pluripotent stem cells (iPSCs) into NSCs and neurons *in vitro,* and promote the survival and neural differentiation of transplanted iPSCs-derived NSCs into the brains of rats with MCAO and function recovery.[96]

Anti-spasmodic Activity

The leaf extract (0.29 mg/kg) from *S. leriifolia* induces skeletal muscle relaxation in mice, being as effective as diazepam (1 mg/kg) which is used for adjunctive treatment for the relief of skeletal muscle spasms due to reflex spasms to local pathology and spasticity caused by upper motor neuron disorders.[97]

Analgesic Activity

The analgesic effect of *S. miltiorrhiza* from root extracts on visceral pain discharge in the posterior nucleus of the thalamus in cats has been assessed using an extracellular microelectrode method and a stereotaxic technique in the brain. *Salvia miltiorrhiza* inhibits the discharge of visceral pain by acting directly on the peripheral nerve trunk via the central nervous system.[98] Another study with the aqueous seed extract of *S. leriifolia* showed a significant anti-nociceptive effect in a dose-dependent (1.25–10 g/kg) manner in the hot-plate test, but not tail flick test which has a spinal mechanism. This effect was inhibited by naloxone pre-treatment, indicating anti-nociceptive effects may be mediated by opioid receptors.[99]

Summary of Pharmacological Actions of the Common Herbs

Each of the ten herbs listed above were contained in formulas in the RCTs and have received great research attention in experimental models of relevance to post-stroke spasticity. Neuroprotective effects against cytotoxicity or death in neurons *in vitro* and against infarction volume and neurological deficit in well-established experimental MCAO-I/R animal models were observed with all extracts or/and their bioactive compounds of herbs except *shen jin cao* 伸筋草. The neuroprotective effect was largely mediated by multiple mechanisms such as antioxidative/nitration stress reaction, anti-inflammatory and anti-apoptotic signalling. However, the number of available studies is limited and a lack of direct evidence exists on the protective activities for both neuronal damage and muscle spasm which exist in post-stroke spasticity patients. Furthermore, investigation with the main compound alone, or combined compounds, in MCAO-I/R post-stroke hypermytonia animal models to clarify the capacity of compound(s) for recovery of damaged motor function and spasticity and disclosing the underlying mechanism(s) is needed.

Anti-spasmodic effect with improved muscle tension and mobility was observed in extracts and/or compounds derived from *bai shao* 白芍, *dang gui* 当归, *mu gua* 木瓜, *gan cao* 甘草, *shen jin cao* 伸筋草, *chuan xiong* 川芎, *huang qi* 黄芪 and *dan shen* 丹参 via modulation of homeostasis of K^{+} and Ca^{2+} channels. Analgesic effects were observed in extracts and/or compounds derived from *bai shao* 白芍,

dang gui 当归, *mu gua* 木瓜, *hong hua* 红花, *chuan xiong* 川芎, *huang qi* 黄芪 and *dan shen* 丹参.

In addition, Chinese herbal medicines have been shown to promote adult neurogenesis; this was also observed in some extracts and/or compounds derived from *dang gui* 当归, *di long* 地龙, *chuan xiong* 川芎 and *dan shen* 丹参. The combination of Chinese herbal medicine and stem cell biology opens a new direction for neuronal regeneration therapy and provides an alternative strategy for post-stroke treatment.[100] The *in vitro* and *in vivo* studies on the post-stroke spasticity-relevant activities, along with more general anti-inflammatory, antioxidant, anti-apoptotic and cardioprotective activities (such as anti-atherogenesis, anti-hyperlipidemic, anti-thrombosis, anti-hypertension and anti-myocardial ischaemia properties) provide potential explanations of the clinical benefits for the herbs contained in the formulas used in the clinical studies of post-stroke spasticity.

References

1. He DY, Dai SM. (2011) Anti-inflammatory and immunomodulatory effects of Paeonia lactiflora Pall., a traditional chinese herbal medicine. *Front Pharmacol* **2:** 10.
2. Parker S, May B, Zhang C, *et al.* (2016) A pharmacological review of bioactive constituents of Paeonia lactiflora Pallas and Paeonia veitchii Lynch. *Phytother Res* **30(9):** 1445–1473.
3. Kim SH, Lee MK, Lee KY, *et al.* (2009) Chemical constituents isolated from Paeonia lactiflora roots and their neuroprotective activity against oxidative stress *in vitro. J Enzyme Inhib Med Chem* **24(5):** 1138–1140.
4. Zhang Y, Qiao L, Xu W, *et al.* (2017) Paeoniflorin attenuates cerebral ischaemia-induced injury by regulating Ca2+/CaMKII/CREB signaling pathway. *Molecules* **22(3):** 359.
5. Liu DZ, Xie KQ, Ji XQ, *et al.* (2005) Neuroprotective effect of paeoniflorin on cerebral ischemic rat by activating adenosine A1 receptor in a manner different from its classical agonists. *Br J Pharmacol* **146(4):** 604–611.
6. Tang NY, Liu CH, Hsieh CT, Hsieh CL. (2010) The anti-inflammatory effect of paeoniflorin on cerebral infarction induced by ischemia-reperfusion injury in Sprague-Dawley rats. *Am J Chin Med* **38(1):** 51–64.

7. Kimura M, Kimura I, Takahashi K, *et al.* (1984) Blocking effects of blended paeoniflorin or its related compounds with glycyrrhizin on neuromuscular junctions in frog and mouse. *Jpn J Pharmacol* **36(3):** 275–282.
8. Zhang H, Yang J, Liu JY, *et al.* (2015) Effect of "Shaoyao Gancao Decoction" on spastic hemiplegia after cerebral ischemia-reperfusion and level of excitatory amino acids in rats. *Shanghai J Tradit Chin Med* **49(5):** 85–89 (article in Chinese, English abstract).
9. Zhang XJ, Chen HL, Li Z, *et al.* (2009) Analgesic effect of paeoniflorin in rats with neonatal maternal separation-induced visceral hyperalgesia is mediated through adenosine A(1) receptor by inhibiting the extracellular signal-regulated protein kinase (ERK) pathway. *Pharmacol Biochem Behav* **94(1):** 88–97.
10. Chao WW, Lin BF. (2011) Bioactivities of major constituents isolated from Angelica sinensis (Danggui). *Chin Med* **6:** 29.
11. Wei WL, Zeng R, Gu CM, *et al.* (2016) Angelica sinensis in China: A review of botanical profile, ethnopharmacology, phytochemistry and chemical analysis. *J Ethnopharmacol* **190:** 116–141.
12. Wu YC, Hsieh CL. (2011) Pharmacological effects of Radix Angelica Sinensis (Danggui) on cerebral infarction. *Chin Med* **6:** 32.
13. Yu Y, Du JR, Wang CY, Qian ZM. (2008) Protection against hydrogen peroxide-induced injury by Z-ligustilide in PC12 cells. *Exp Brain Res* **184(3):** 307–312.
14. Cheng CY, Ho TY, Lee EJ, *et al.* (2008) Ferulic acid reduces cerebral infarct through its antioxidative and anti-inflammatory effects following transient focal cerebral ischemia in rats. *Am J Chin Med* **36(6):** 1105–1119.
15. Peng HY, Du JR, Zhang GY, *et al.* (2007) Neuroprotective effect of Z-ligustilide against permanent focal ischemic damage in rats. *Biol Pharm Bull* **30(2):** 309–312.
16. Kuang X, Yao Y, Du JR, *et al.* (2006) Neuroprotective role of Z-ligustilide against forebrain ischemic injury in ICR mice. *Brain Res* **1102(1):** 145–153.
17. Kuang X, Du JR, Liu YX, *et al.* (2008) Postischemic administration of Z-Ligustilide ameliorates cognitive dysfunction and brain damage induced by permanent forebrain ischemia in rats. *Pharmacol Biochem Behav* **88(3):** 213–221.
18. Xin J, Zhang J, Yang Y, *et al.* (2013) Radix Angelica Sinensis that contains the component Z-ligustilide promotes adult neurogenesis to

mediate recovery from cognitive impairment. *Curr Neurovasc Res* **10(4):** 304–315.
19. Zhang Q, Zhao Y, Xu Y, *et al.* (2016) Sodium ferulate and n-butylidenephthalate combined with bone marrow stromal cells (BMSCs) improve the therapeutic effects of angiogenesis and neurogenesis after rat focal cerebral ischemia. *J Transl Med* **14(1):** 223.
20. Ko WC. (1980) A newly isolated antispasmodic: Butylidenephthalide. *Jpn J Pharmacol* **30(1):** 85–91.
21. Song M, Li Q, He C. (2009) Identification and analgetic effect of Angelica sinensis extract. *J Xianning Univ* **23:** 194–196.
22. Du H, Wu J, Li H, *et al.* (2013) Polyphenols and triterpenes from Chaenomeles fruits: Chemical analysis and antioxidant activities assessment. *Food Chem* **141(4):** 4260–4268.
23. Zhang SY, Han LY, Zhang H, Xin HL. (2014) Chaenomeles speciosa: A review of chemistry and pharmacology. *Biomed Rep* **2(1):** 12–18.
24. Rong ZT, Gong XJ, Sun HB, *et al.* (2011) Protective effects of oleanolic acid on cerebral ischemic damage in vivo and H(2)O(2)-induced injury in vitro. *Pharm Biol* **49(1):** 78–85.
25. Ning Y, Huang J, Kalionis B, *et al.* (2015) Oleanolic acid induces differentiation of neural stem cells to neurons: An involvement of transcription factor Nkx-2.5. *Stem Cells Int* **2015:** 672312.
26. Li L, Zhang X, Cui L, *et al.* (2013) Ursolic acid promotes the neuroprotection by activating Nrf2 pathway after cerebral ischemia in mice. *Brain Res* **1497:** 32–39.
27. Wang H, Li SY, Zhao CK, Zeng X. (2009) A system for screening agonists targeting β2 adrenoceptor from Chinese medicinal herbs. *J Zhejiang Univ Sci B* **10:** 243–250.
28. Kong JS, Yang XH, Liu W. (2007) The relaxant effects and related mechanism of total flavones from Chaenomeles lagenaria Koidz on gastrointestinal smooth muscles. *Lishizhen Med Mater Med Res* **18:** 2123–2124.
29. Liu W, Yang XH, Zhou M, Li CD. (2007) Pharmacodynamical mechanisms of total flavonoids from Chaenomeles lagenaria Koidz in the relaxation of gastrointestinal smooth muscles. *World Chin J Digestol* **15:** 165–167.
30. Wang NP, Dai M, Wang H, *et al.* (2005) Antinociceptive effect of glucosides of Chaenomeles speciosa. *Chin J Pharmacol Toxicol* **19:** 169–174.
31. Li X, Yang YB, Yang Q, *et al.* (2009) Anti-inflammatory and analgesic activities of Chaenomeles speciosa fractions in laboratory animals. *J Med Food* **12(5):** 1016–1022.

32. Asl MN, Hosseinzadeh H. (2008) Review of pharmacological effects of Glycyrrhiza sp. and its bioactive compounds. *Phytother Res* **22(6):** 709–724.
33. Ji S, Li Z, Song W, *et al.* (2016) Bioactive constituents of Glycyrrhiza uralensis (licorice): Discovery of the effective components of a traditional herbal medicine. *J Nat Prod* **79(2):** 281–292.
34. Zhang Q, Ye M. (2009) Chemical analysis of the Chinese herbal medicine Gan-Cao (licorice). *J Chromatogr A* **1216(11):** 1954–1969.
35. Peng F, Du Q, Peng C, *et al.* (2015) A review: The pharmacology of isoliquiritigenin. *Phytother Res* **29(7):** 969–977.
36. Yang EJ, Min JS, Ku HY, *et al.* (2012) Isoliquiritigenin isolated from Glycyrrhiza uralensis protects neuronal cells against glutamate-induced mitochondrial dysfunction. *Biochem Biophys Res Commun* **421(4):** 658–664.
37. Lee HK, Yang EJ, Kim JY, *et al.* (2012) Inhibitory effects of Glycyrrhizae radix and its active component, isoliquiritigenin, on Aβ(25–35)-induced neurotoxicity in cultured rat cortical neurons. *Arch Pharm Res* **35(5):** 897–904.
38. Zhan, C, Yang J. (2006) Protective effects of isoliquiritigenin in transient middle cerebral artery occlusion-induced focal cerebral ischemia in rats. *Pharmacol Res* **53(3):** 303–309.
39. Sun YX, Tang Y, Wu AL, *et al.* (2010) Neuroprotective effect of liquiritin against focal cerebral ischemia/reperfusion in mice via its antioxidant and antiapoptosis properties. *J Asian Nat Prod Res* **12(12):** 1051–1060.
40. Zhang LL, Tian K, Tang ZH, *et al.* (2016) Phytochemistry and pharmacology of Carthamus tinctorius L. *Am J Chin Med* **44(2):** 197–226.
41. Zhou X, Tang L, Xu Y, *et al.* (2014) Towards a better understanding of medicinal uses of Carthamus tinctorius L. in traditional Chinese medicine: A phytochemical and pharmacological review. *J Ethnopharmacol* **151(1):** 27–43.
42. Yang Q, Yang ZF, Liu SB, *et al.* (2010) Neuroprotective effects of hydroxysafflor yellow A against excitotoxic neuronal death partially through down-regulation of NR2B-containing NMDA receptors. *Neurochem Res* **35(9):** 1353–1360.
43. Kong SZ, Xian YF, Ip SP, *et al.* (2013) Protective effects of hydroxysafflor yellow A on beta-amyloid-induced neurotoxicity in PC12 cells. *Neurochem Res* **38(5):** 951–960.

44. Zhu HB, Zhang L, Wang ZH, *et al.* (2005) Therapeutic effects of hydroxysafflor yellow A on focal cerebral ischemic injury in rats and its primary mechanisms. *J Asian Nat Prod Res* **7(4):** 607–613.
45. Chen L, Xiang Y, Kong L, *et al.* (2013) Hydroxysafflor yellow A protects against cerebral ischemia-reperfusion injury by anti-apoptotic effect through PI3K/Akt/GSK3beta pathway in rat. *Neurochem Res* **38(11):** 2268–2275.
46. Sun L, Yang L, Fu Y, *et al.* (2013) Capacity of HSYA to inhibit nitrotyrosine formation induced by focal ischemic brain injury. *Nitric Oxide* **35:** 144–151.
47. Fu PK, Pan TL, Yang CY, *et al.* (2016) Carthamus tinctorius L. ameliorates brain injury followed by cerebral ischemia-reperfusion in rats by antioxidative and anti-inflammatory mechanisms. *Iran J Basic Med Sci* **19(12):** 1368–1375.
48. Yu L, Chen C, Wang LF, *et al.* (2013) Neuroprotective effect of kaempferol glycosides against brain injury and neuroinflammation by inhibiting the activation of NF-kappaB and STAT3 in transient focal stroke. *PLoS One* **8(2):** e55839.
49. Huang ZL, Yu ML, Qu SK, *et al.* (1984) Studies on the immuno-activity of the polysaccharide from safflower (Carthamus tinectorius). *Chin Trad Herb Drugs* **15:** 213–216.
50. Popov AM, Li IA, Kang DI. (2009) Analgesic properties of CF extracted from the Safflor (Carthamus tinctorius) seeds and its potential uses. *Pharm Chem J* **43(1):** 41–44.
51. Wu J, Wang H, Ma Y, *et al.* (2015) Isolation of a new lycodine alkaloid from Lycopodium japonicum. *Nat Prod Res* **29(8):** 735–738.
52. He J, Wu XD, Liu F, *et al.* (2014) Lycopodine-type alkaloids from Lycopodium japonicum. *Nat Prod Bioprospect* **4(4):** 213–219.
53. Sun ZH, Li W, Tang GH, Yin S. (2017) A new serratene triterpenoid from Lycopodium japonicum. *J Asian Nat Prod Res* **19(3):** 299–303.
54. Wang XJ, Li L, Yu SS, *et al.* (2013) Five new fawcettimine-related alkaloids from Lycopodium japonicum Thunb. *Fitoterapia* **91:** 74–81.
55. Yang Q, Zhu Y, Peng W, *et al.* (2016) A new lycopodine-type alkaloid from Lycopodium japonicum. *Nat Prod Res* **30(19):** 2220–2224.
56. Konrath EL, Ortega MG, de Loreto Bordignon S, *et al.* (2013) Alkaloid profiling and anticholinesterase activity of South American Lycopodiaceae species. *J Enzyme Inhib Med Chem* **28(1):** 218–222.

57. Ortega MG, Agnese AM, Cabrera JL. (2004) Anticholinesterase activity in an alkaloid extract of Huperzia saururus. *Phytomedicine* **11(6):** 539–543.
58. Konrath EL, Neves BM, Passos Cdos S, *et al.* (2012) Huperzia quadrifariata and Huperzia reflexa alkaloids inhibit acetylcholinesterase activity in vivo in mice brain. *Phytomedicine* **19(14):** 1321–1324.
59. Cooper EL, Balamurugan M, Huang CY, *et al.* (2012) Earthworms dilong: Ancient, inexpensive, noncontroversial models may help clarify approaches to integrated medicine emphasizing neuroimmune systems. *Evid Based Complement Alternat Med* **2012:** 164152.
60. Wang G, Hu D, Chen J, *et al.* (1998) Analysis of chemical components from Pheretima. *J Chin Med Mater* **21(3):** 133–135.
61. Chang YM, Kuo WH, Lai TY, *et al.* (2011) RSC96 schwann cell proliferation and survival induced by Dilong through PI3K/Akt signaling mediated by IGF-I. *Evid Based Complement Alternat Med* **2011:** 216148.
62. Chang YM, Shih YT, Chen YS, *et al.* (2011) Schwann cell migration induced by earthworm extract via activation of PAs and MMP2/9 mediated through ERK1/2 and p38. *Evid Based Complement Alternat Med* **2011:** 395458.
63. Chen CT, Lin JG, Lu TW, *et al.* (2010) Earthworm extracts facilitate PC12 cell differentiation and promote axonal sprouting in peripheral nerve injury. *Am J Chin Med* **38(3):** 547–560.
64. Liu CH, Lin YW, Tang NY, *et al.* (2012) Effect of oral administration of Pheretima aspergillum (earthworm) in rats with cerebral infarction induced by middle-cerebral artery occlusion. *Afr J Tradit Complement Altern Med* **10(1):** 66–82.
65. Ji H, Wang L, Bi H, *et al.* (2008) Mechanisms of lumbrokinase in protection of cerebral ischemia. *Eur J Pharmacol* **590(1–3):** 281–289.
66. Kim DH, Lee IH, Nam ST, *et al.* (2014) Neurotropic and neuroprotective activities of the earthworm peptide Lumbricusin. *Biochem Biophys Res Commun* **448(3):** 292–297.
67. Kim DH, Lee IH, Nam ST, *et al.* (2015) Antimicrobial peptide, lumbricusin, ameliorates motor dysfunction and dopaminergic neurodegeneration in a mouse model of Parkinson's disease. *J Microbiol Biotechnol* **25(10):** 1640–1647.
68. Seo M, Lee JH, Baek M, *et al.* (2017) A novel role for earthworm peptide Lumbricusin as a regulator of neuroinflammation. *Biochem Biophys Res Commun* **490(3):** 1004–1010.

69. Li W, Tang Y, Chen Y, Duan JA. (2012) Advances in the chemical analysis and biological activities of chuanxiong. *Molecules* **17(9):** 10614–10651.
70. Ran X, Ma L, Peng C, *et al.* (2011) Ligusticum chuanxiong Hort: A review of chemistry and pharmacology. *Pharm Biol* **49(11):** 1180–1189.
71. Wu XM, Qian ZM, Zhu L, *et al.* (2011) Neuroprotective effect of ligustilide against ischaemia-reperfusion injury via up-regulation of erythropoietin and down-regulation of RTP801. *Br J Pharmacol* **164(2):** 332–343.
72. Chen Z, Pan X, Georgakilas AG, *et al.* (2013) Tetramethylpyrazine (TMP) protects cerebral neurocytes and inhibits glioma by down regulating chemokine receptor CXCR4 expression. *Cancer Lett* **336(2):** 281–289.
73. Li SY, Jia YH, Sun WG, *et al.* (2010) Stabilization of mitochondrial function by tetramethylpyrazine protects against kainate-induced oxidative lesions in the rat hippocampus. *Free Radic Biol Med* **48(4):** 597–608.
74. Kao TK, Chang CY, Ou YC, *et al.* (2013) Tetramethylpyrazine reduces cellular inflammatory response following permanent focal cerebral ischemia in rats. *Exp Neurol* **247:** 188–201.
75. Wu W, Yu X, Luo XP, *et al.* (2013) Tetramethylpyrazine protects against scopolamine-induced memory impairments in rats by reversing the cAMP/PKA/CREB pathway. *Behav Brain Res* **253:** 212–216.
76. Xiao X, Liu Y, Qi C, *et al.* (2010) Neuroprotection and enhanced neurogenesis by tetramethylpyrazine in adult rat brain after focal ischemia. *Neurol Res* **32(5):** 547–555.
77. Tian Y, Liu Y, Chen X, *et al.* (2010) Tetramethylpyrazine promotes proliferation and differentiation of neural stem cells from rat brain in hypoxic condition via mitogen-activated protein kinases pathway *in vitro*. *Neurosci Lett* **474(1):** 26–31.
78. Yan Y, Zhao J, Cao C, *et al.* (2014) Tetramethylpyrazine promotes SH-SY5Y cell differentiation into neurons through epigenetic regulation of Topoisomerase IIβ. *Neuroscience* **278:**179–193.
79. Ozaki Y, Sekita S, Harada M. (1989) Centrally acting muscle relaxant effect of phthalides (ligustilide, cnidilide and senkyunolide) obtained from Cnidium officinale Makino [article in Japanese]. *Yakugaku Zasshi* **109(6):** 402–406.

80. Bie BH, Chen Y, Zhao ZQ. (2006) Ligustrazine inhibits high voltage-gated Ca(2+) and TTX-resistant Na(+) channels of primary sensory neuron and thermal nociception in the rat: A study on peripheral mechanism. *Neurosci Bull* **22(2):** 79–84.
81. Fu J, Wang Z, Huang L, *et al.* (2014) Review of the botanical characteristics, phytochemistry, and pharmacology of Astragalus membranaceus (Huangqi). *Phytother Res* **28(9):** 1275–1283.
82. Li X, Qu L, Dong Y, *et al.* (2014) A review of recent research progress on the Astragalus genus. *Molecules* **19(11):** 18850–18880.
83. Li L, Hou X, Xu R, *et al.* (2017) Research review on the pharmacological effects of astragaloside IV. *Fundam Clin Pharmacol* **31(1):** 17–36.
84. Wang HL, Zhou QH, Xu MB, *et al.* (2017) Astragaloside IV for experimental focal cerebral ischemia: Preclinical evidence and possible mechanisms. *Oxid Med Cell Longev* **2017:** 8424326.
85. Gao J, Liu ZJ, Chen T, Zhao D. (2014) Pharmaceutical properties of calycosin, the major bioactive isoflavonoid in the dry root extract of Radix astragali. *Pharm Biol* **52(9):** 1217–1222.
86. Guo C, Tong L, Xi M, *et al.* (2012) Neuroprotective effect of calycosin on cerebral ischemia and reperfusion injury in rats. *J Ethnopharmacol* **144(3):** 768–774.
87. Guo C, Ma Y, Ma S, *et al.* (2017) The role of TRPC6 in the neuroprotection of calycosin against cerebral ischemic injury. *Sci Rep* **7(1):** 3039.
88. Wu XL, Wang YY, Cheng J, Zhao YY. (2006) Calcium channel blocking activity of calycosin, a major active component of Astragali Radix, on rat aorta. *Acta Pharmacol Sin* **27(8):** 1007–1012.
89. Revuelta MP, Cantabrana B, Hidalgo A. (2000) Mechanisms involved in kaempferol-induced relaxation in rat uterine smooth muscle. *Life Sci* **67(3):** 251–259.
90. Su CY, Ming QL, Rahman K, *et al.* (2015) Salvia miltiorrhiza: Traditional medicinal uses, chemistry, and pharmacology. *Chin J Nat Med* **13(3):** 163–182.
91. Wang BQ. (2010) Salvia miltiorrhiza: Chemical and pharmacological review of a medicinal plant. *J Med Plant Res* **4:** 2813–2820.
92. Imanshahidi M, Hosseinzadeh H. (2006) The pharmacological effects of Salvia species on the central nervous system. *Phytother Res* **20(6):** 427–437.
93. Bonaccini L, Karioti A, Bergonzi MC, Bilia AR. (2015) Effects of Salvia miltiorrhiza on CNS neuronal injury and degeneration: A plausible

complementary role of tanshinones and depsides. *Planta Med* **81(12–13):** 1003–1016.

94. Zhuang P, Zhang Y, Cui G, *et al.* (2012) Direct stimulation of adult neural stem/progenitor cells *in vitro* and neurogenesis *in vivo* by salvianolic acid B. *PLoS One* **7(4):** e35636.
95. Zhang N, Kang T, Xia Y, *et al.* (2012) Effects of salvianolic acid B on survival, self-renewal and neuronal differentiation of bone marrow derived neural stem cells. *Eur J Pharmacol* **697(1–3):** 32–39.
96. Shu T, Pang M, Rong L, *et al.* (2014) Effects of Salvia miltiorrhiza on neural differentiation of induced pluripotent stem cells. *J Ethnopharmacol* **153(1):** 233–241.
97. Hosseinzadeh H, Hassanzadeh AR. (2001) Muscle relaxant and hypnotic effects of Salvia leriifolia Benth. leaves extract in mice. *Iran J Basic Med Sci* **4:** 130–138.
98. Liu C, Shi W, Sun L, Zheng Q. (1990) Effects of radix Salviae miltiorrhizae on visceral pain discharges in the posterior nucleus of the thalamus in cats [In Chinese]. *Zhongguo Zhong Yao Za Zhi* **15:** 112–115.
99. Hosseinzadeh H, Haddadkhodaparast MH, Arash AR. (2003) Antinociceptive, antiinflammatory and acute toxicity effects of Salvia leriifolia Benth seed extract in mice and rats. *Phytother Res* **17(4):** 422–425.
100. Shen J, Chen X, Chen X, Deng R. (2014) Targeting neurogenesis: A promising therapeutic strategy for post-stroke treatment with Chinese herbal medicine. *Integr Med Int* **1:** 5–18.

7

Clinical Evidence for Acupuncture and Related Therapies

OVERVIEW

Acupuncture therapies are commonly researched in clinical studies for post-stroke spasticity. Extensive searches of nine electronic databases identified almost 30,000 citations for the condition. One hundred and fifty-one randomised controlled trials, 12 controlled clinical trials and 35 non-controlled studies were included in this chapter. The results showed that the evidence of acupuncture therapies was promising. In particular, when acupuncture therapies were used as add-on therapy to routine care/rehabilitation, they were effective for spasticity severity, motor function and the activities of daily living.

Introduction

Acupuncture is a common technique to treat disease by correcting imbalances and restoring health. Methods of stimulating acupuncture points include:

- Acupuncture: Insertion of an acupuncture needle into acupuncture points;
- Acupressure: Application of pressure to acupuncture points;
- Moxibustion: Burning of a herb (usually *ai ye* 艾叶, *Artemesia vulgaris* L.) close to, or on, the skin to induce a warming sensation;
- Electroacupuncture: Electric stimulation of the needle following insertion.

Whilst many of these therapies have ancient roots, several have emerged as new techniques in the last century. These include scalp acupuncture 头皮针 and wrist-ankle acupuncture 腕踝针.

- Scalp acupuncture 头皮针: Acupuncture micro-system at the specific lines located on the scalp;
- Wrist-ankle acupuncture 腕踝针: Acupuncture micro-system at the points located at wrist and ankle.

Previous Systematic Reviews

The efficacy and safety of acupuncture-related therapies for post-stroke spasticity have been systematically reviewed by two publications in English.[1,2] Both systematic reviews included studies of manual acupuncture and electroacupuncture. Modified Ashworth Scale (MAS), the main outcome measure for spasticity, was evaluated by meta-analysis in both systematic reviews.[1,2]

Park *et al.* (2014)[1] systematically reviewed eight randomised controlled trials (RCTs) published between 2001 and 2008, with 399 participants. Interventions were manual acupuncture (n = 3) and electroacupuncture (n = 5), while the controls used were sham acupuncture (n = 1) or conventional rehabilitation (n = 7). Meta-analysis showed that, compared with controls using conventional rehabilitation (without acupuncture), acupuncture had no effect on improving clinical outcomes (as measured by validated instruments such as MAS) or physiologic outcomes (assessed by measures such as the H-reflex/M-response ratio at the end of the treatment period). The H-reflex/M-response ratio did decrease significantly immediately after the first acupuncture treatment. This review concluded that the effect of acupuncture for post-stroke spasticity remains uncertain, mainly because of the poor quality of the available studies.

Lim *et al.* (2015)[2] searched English and Chinese databases, as well as 19 Korean journals, to July 2013. Five RCTs were included in this review; of them, three were published in English, one in Korean and one in Chinese. One RCT compared acupuncture to sham acupuncture, one compared the combination of acupuncture and standard therapy with standard therapy alone, and another three RCTs compared the combination of electroacupuncture and standard therapy with standard therapy alone. Assessments were performed primarily with MAS. Meta-analysis showed that acupuncture or electroacupuncture significantly decreased spasticity after stroke. Subgroup analysis showed that acupuncture significantly decreased wrist, knee and elbow spasticity in post-stroke patients. Heterogeneity could be explained by the differences in control and acupoints, and the duration after stroke occurrence. A conclusion was drawn by the authors that acupuncture could be effective in decreasing spasticity after stroke, but long-term studies are needed to determine the longevity of treatment effects.

Identification of Clinical Studies

A total of 37,141 citations were identified after searching Chinese and English databases. A total of 198 studies were included in this chapter, with 151 RCTs (A1–A151), 12 controlled clinical trials (CCTs, A152–A163), and 35 non-controlled studies (A164–A198) (Fig. 1).

All of the included studies were conducted in China, except one study conducted in Germany (A1). Over 13,000 participants were observed in these studies. Evidence from RCTs and CCTs was pooled to evaluate the efficacy and safety of acupuncture therapies. Results from non-controlled studies were only described for the main characteristics. A number of acupuncture therapies were investigated by these studies. They are body acupuncture, scalp acupuncture, electroacupuncture, transcutaneous electrical nerve stimulation (TENS), moxibustion, acupressure, and their combinations. In addition, 11 studies investigated acupuncture interventions not commonly practised outside of China; they will not be presented here.

A total of over 12,000 participants were included in the 151 RCTs (A1–A151). The average age of participants was 60.5 years. Of the studies which reported information on participants' gender, there were more males (n = 6,256) than females (n = 4,314).

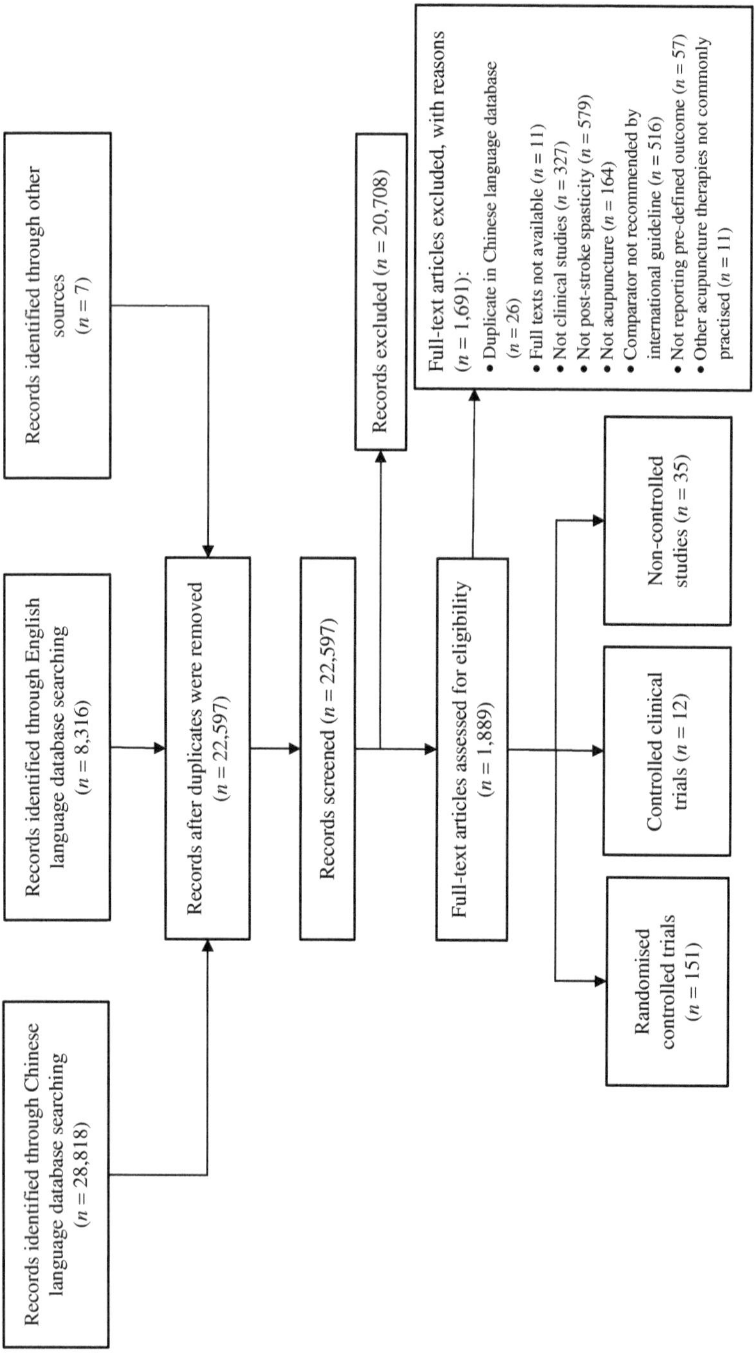

Fig. 7.1 Flowchart of study selection process: acupuncture and related therapies.

The treatment duration ranged from two weeks (A4, A11, A12, A19, A20–A22) to three months (A23–A27). Eight studies (A9, A13, A16–A18, A28–A30) reported information of participants' syndromes. The most common syndrome seen in these studies is 'Liver *yang* uprising, Wind and Phlegm blocking the meridians, with *qi* deficiency and Blood stasis'. A number of acupuncture-related interventions were evaluated by these RCTs, including body acupuncture, scalp acupuncture, electroacupuncture, TENs, moxibustion, acupressure, and their combinations.

An acupuncture technique named *Jin San Zhen* 靳三针 has been evaluated in 16 RCTs (A3–A18). *Jin San Zhen* 靳三针 is an acupuncture treatment theory created by Professor Rui Jin, including a total of 23 different needling techniques for treating different clinical conditions. Among them, needling the temporal area with three needles (颞三针) is usually used for post-stroke hemiplegia. However, these 16 studies did not limit their acupuncture treatments to the temporal area with three needles (颞三针); other body points commonly used for stroke were also selected. Hence these studies could not be considered as a subgroup in our evaluation.

Among the 151 included RCTs, 116 studies were two-armed studies, with 24 of them comparing acupuncture therapies with different comparators and 92 studies assessing the add-on effects of acupuncture therapies to different comparators. Twenty-three RCTs were three-armed studies which contained both the abovementioned comparisons. Two studies (A26, A136) were three-armed studies, with only two arms evaluating the add-on effects of acupuncture therapies and meeting our inclusion criteria. The remaining ten RCTs were three-armed studies containing two acupuncture groups; one used a special acupuncture technique and another one used routine acupuncture treatment as control. For these ten studies, the treatment effects of the special acupuncture technique were analysed for efficacy evaluation, with six of them evaluating the add-on effects. Overall, acupuncture therapies were compared to placebo or sham needling ($n = 2$), Western medicine drugs or routine care/rehabilitation ($n = 47$) and electrical stimulation ($n = 1$). The add-on effects of acupuncture therapies integrated with other treatments were assessed in a total of 123 RCTs.

In total, over 170 body acupuncture points were used by the included studies; the most commonly selected points were LI4 *Hegu* 合谷 (*n* = 39), LI11 *Quchi* 曲池 (*n* = 38), TE5 *Waiguan* 外关 (*n* = 36), SP6 *Sanyinjiao* 三阴交 (*n* = 32), LI15 *Jianyu* 肩髃 (*n* = 27), LI10 *Shousanli* 手三里 (*n* = 26), GB34 *Yanglingquan* 阳陵泉 (*n* = 25), SP9 *Yinlingquan* 阴陵泉 (*n* = 24), ST36 *Zusanli* 足三里 (*n* = 24), LU5 *Chize* 尺泽 (*n* = 24), PC6 *Neiguan* 内关 (*n* = 20), HT1 *Jiquan* 极泉 (*n* = 20), SP10 *Xuehai* 血海 (*n* = 17), KI6 *Zhaohai* 照海 (*n* = 17), LR3 *Taichong* 太冲 (*n* = 15), GB40 *Qiuxu* 丘墟 (*n* = 15), BL40 *Weizhong* 委中 (*n* = 15), GV20 *Baihui* 百会 (*n* = 12), ST41 *Jiexi* 解溪 (*n* = 12) and BL37 *Yinmen* 殷门 (*n* = 11). In addition to these body acupuncture points, scalp acupuncture was also applied on different treatment zones.

Risk of Bias Assessment

Included studies were described as 'randomised' but only 69 studies introduced the correct methods for sequence generation. Twelve studies which used sealed envelopes for allocation concealment were judged as 'low' risk; 139 studies did not describe the details, therefore were 'unclear' risk. Blinding of participants was performed in two single-blinded studies by adapting a placebo/sham control method; therefore these two studies were 'low' risk for this item, while the other 149 were judged as 'high' risk. Blinding of personnel was not seen in any of these studies; hence they were all of 'high' risk for this item. Seven studies made an effort in blinding the outcome assessors; the remaining studies were judged to be 'unclear' risk for this. All studies were 'low' risk for incomplete outcome data because there was no high drop-out rate. For the selective reporting, all studies were judged as 'unclear' risk as the protocols were not published or registered with clinical trial registration. See Table 7.1 for a summary.

Outcomes

The commonly reported outcome measures of the included studies were Ashworth Scale (AS), MAS, Fugl-Meyer Assessment (FMA) and

Table 7.1 Risk of Bias of Randomised Controlled Trials: All Acupuncture Therapies

Risk of Bias Domain	Low Risk *n* (%)	Unclear Risk *n* (%)	High Risk *n* (%)
Sequence generation	69 (45.7)	78 (51.7)	4 (2.6)
Allocation concealment	12 (7.9)	139 (92.1)	0 (0)
Blinding of participants	2 (1.3)	0 (0)	149 (98.7)
Blinding of personnel	0 (0)	0 (0)	151 (100)
Blinding of outcome assessors	7 (4.6)	144 (95.4)	0 (0)
Incomplete outcome data	151 (100)	0 (0)	0 (0)
Selective outcome reporting	0 (0)	151 (100)	0 (0)

Blinding of personnel (acupuncturists) is challenging in manual therapies.

Barthel Index (BI). Being the primary outcome for spasticity, data of AS or MAS were reported in 96 studies. Among them, 55 studies reported scores of AS or MAS, while another 41 studies reported how many participants were assessed as each level of AS or MAS; these data were then converted to scores for further data analyses. Ashworth Scale or MAS was reported to evaluate the spasticity of unspecified regions, upper limb, lower limb, different joints or muscles. Meta-analysis was conducted for the data of AS or MAS for unspecified region, upper limb and lower limb. It is noted that AS or MAS was measured using different scales including [0, 1, 1.5, 2, 3, 4], [0, 1, 2, 3, 4, 5] and [1, 2, 3, 4, 5, 6]; therefore data of these scores were presented using standardised mean difference (SMD) in our meta-analysis.

Acupuncture therapies' effects of the main outcomes are summarised below within each category of intervention and comparator.

Acupuncture

Randomised Controlled Trials of Acupuncture

Acupuncture versus Sham Acupuncture (Sham Needling)

Two studies (A1, A31) compared acupuncture to sham needling methods. Fink *et al.* (2004) (A1) employed blunt needles on non-acupoints, and Li *et al.* (2013) (A31) used short needles with a superficial needling on non-acupoints as the sham control method.

Modified Ashworth Scale

Both studies (A1, A31) reported data on MAS without stating the measurement/calculation method. The MAS scores reported by one study involving 138 participants (A31) seem incorrect (e.g., acupuncture: 23.98 ± 10.84; control: 21.87 ± 9.46; these scores are outside of the normal range of MAS) and this study did not explain what criteria were used for measuring. The other study (A1) showed there was no difference between the acupuncture and sham control (mean difference (MD): 0.00 [–0.79, 0.79]), with a very small sample size (acupuncture: 13 versus control: 12).

Fugl-Myer Assessment

Li *et al.* (A31) reported data on FMA (motor) at the end-of-treatment and follow-up phases. No significant difference between the real and sham acupuncture was found for this outcome after a four-week treatment (MD: 4.50 [–1.33, 10.33]); on the other hand, a significant difference was shown at the end of the follow-up phase (MD: 11.48 [5.68, 17.28]).

Barthel Index

The BI data at the end-of-treatment and follow-up phases were also reported by Li *et al.* (A31). Similar to the results for FMA, it was found that there was no significant difference between the real and sham acupuncture at the end-of-treatment phase (MD: 0.21 [–5.19, 5.61]); however, a significant difference was shown at the end of the follow-up phase (MD: 10.00 [4.54, 15.46]).

Due to the small number of studies ($n = 2$) comparing real acupuncture to sham control, conclusions could not be drawn.

Acupuncture versus Pharmacotherapy

Six studies compared acupuncture with pharmacotherapy; all of them used routine care and rehabilitation as co-interventions (A32–A34, A36, A37, A48). The pharmacotherapy drugs used as comparators were baclofen (A32, A33, A37, A48), piracetam (A34) and MYONAL® (A36). The results of meta-analyses are presented in Table 7.2.

Table 7.2 Meta-analyses Results: Acupuncture (at the End of Treatment)

Comparison	Outcome	No. of Studies	No. of Participants	Effect Size [95% CI]	I^2 (%)	Included Studies
Acupuncture versus pharmacotherapies	AS or MAS (upper limb)	4	697	SMD: −1.20 [−2.12, −0.28]*	95	A34, A36, A37, A48
	FMA (motor)	2	140	MD: 13.35 [−11.29, 37.99]	100	A32, A36
	FMA (upper limb)	3	548	MD: 5.31 [2.85, 7.77]*	100	A33, A34
Acupuncture versus routine care/rehabilitation	AS or MAS (unspecified)	6	403	SMD: −0.18 [−0.58, 0.21]	74	A41–A43, A50, A53, A55
	FMA (motor)	14	1,041	MD: 6.16 [0.41, 11.91]*	95	A4, A10–A13, A17, A18, A25, A28, A41, A42, A54, A57, A72
	FMA (upper limb)	7	616	MD: 0.64 [−3.33, 4.60]	82	A5, A16–A18, A46, A50, A56
	FMA (lower limb)	4	336	MD −1.23 [−6.42, 3.95]	92	A5, A16, A18, A44
	BI or MBI	16	1,356	MD: 8.39 [−1.24, 18.01]	99	A5, A6, A10, A16–A18, A25, A28, A49, A53–A55, A57, A72, A84, A104

*Statistically significant.

Abbreviations: AS – Ashworth Scale; BI – Barthel Index; CI – confidence interval; FMA – Fugl-Meyer Assessment; MAS – Modified Ashworth Scale; MBI – Modified Barthel Index; MD – mean difference; SMD – standardised mean difference.

Modified Ashworth Scale

All six studies (A32–A34, A36, A37, A48) reported data on MAS, with two studies (A32, A33) reporting MAS scores of four individual joints, three studies (A34, A36, A37) reporting upper limb MAS scores and one study not specifying MAS scores (A48). Meta-analysis showed that acupuncture treatment achieved better effects than pharmacotherapies for MAS (upper limb) (SMD: –1.20 [–2.12, –0.28], $I^2 = 95\%$) (A34, A36, A37, A48).

Fugl-Myer Assessment

Two studies (A32, A36) reported FMA (motor); there was no significant difference between acupuncture and pharmacotherapies (MD: 13.35 [–11.29, 37.99], $I^2 = 100\%$); however, very high heterogeneity was detected. Two studies (A33, A34) reported data on FMA (upper limb); a significant difference between the two groups was found (MD: 5.31 [2.85, 7.77], $I^2 = 0\%$). Only one study (A33) reported data on the FMA (lower limb) score at the end-of-treatment phase, without any significant difference between the two groups (MD: 3.46 [–0.69, 7.61]).

Barthel Index

One study (A37) reported data on BI, which detected that the effects of acupuncture were superior to pharmacotherapy (MD: 13.75 [8.84, 18.66]).

Acupuncture versus Routine Care/Rehabilitation

A total of 31 studies compared acupuncture with routine care and rehabilitation; 16 of these were two-armed studies (A6, A10, A13, A25, A28, A39–A46, A72, A84, A104). The other 15 studies (A4, A5, A11, A12, A16–A18, A49, A50, A52–A57) were three-armed studies which included three groups: acupuncture, routine care/rehabilitation, and acupuncture plus routine care/rehabilitation. Treatment effects are presented for each outcome below. The results of meta-analyses are presented in Table 7.2.

Ashworth Scale or Modified Ashworth Scale

One study (A57) reported incorrect data of MAS; therefore it was not included in our analysis. For AS or MAS (unspecified), meta-analysis of six studies (A41–A43, A50, A53, A55) showed that there was no significant difference between acupuncture treatment and routine care/rehabilitation (SMD: –0.18 [–0.58, 0.21], I^2 = 74%). For AS or MAS (upper limb), results of a single study (A56) showed no difference between acupuncture and routine care/rehabilitation (MD: –0.25 [–0.75, 0.25]).

Fugl-Myer Assessment

Fourteen studies (A4, A10–A13, A17, A18, A25, A28, A41, A42, A54, A57, A72) reported data on FMA (motor). Meta-analysis showed that acupuncture was superior to routine care/rehabilitation at the end-of-treatment phase (MD: 6.16 [0.41, 11.91], I^2 = 95%). Two studies (A12, A72) reported data from the end of a follow-up phase on FMA (motor) with no significant difference being found (MD: 20.35 [–14.46, 55.16], I^2 = 99%).

For the FMA scores of upper limb (A5, A16–A18, A46, A50, A56) and FMA scores of lower limb (A5, A16, A18, A44), meta-analyses results also suggested there was no significant difference between acupuncture and the routine care/rehabilitation (FMA upper limb: MD: 0.64 [–3.33, 4.60], I^2 = 82%; FMA lower limb: MD: –1.23 [–6.42, 3.95], I^2 = 94%).

Barthel Index

A total of 16 studies (A5, A6, A10, A16–A18, A25, A28, A49, A53–A55, A57, A72, A84, A104) reported end-of-treatment data on BI or modified BI (MBI). Meta-analysis showed that there was no difference between acupuncture and routine care/rehabilitation for this outcome (MD: 8.39 [–1.24, 18.01], I^2 = 99%).

Acupuncture versus Electrical Stimulation

One study (A58) compared acupuncture with electrostimulation (Hufschmidt's therapy). Both groups also received routine rehabilitation as co-intervention. Treatment was applied for three weeks for both groups. Post-treatment data of MAS (upper limb), FMA (upper limb) and MBI outcomes were reported. Treatment effects were in favour of acupuncture for MBI (MD: 11.67 [4.19, 19.15]); however, not for MAS (upper limb) (MD: –0.18 [–0.66, 0.30]) or FMA (upper limb) (MD: 6.50 [–2.63, 15.63]).

One study (A116) compared scalp acupuncture with Motomed, a motor driven, software-controlled movement therapy unit. After one-month's treatment, the post-treatment data of FMA (lower limb) (MD: –0.30 [–2.75, 2.15]) and BI (MD: –0.25 [–3.22, 2.72]) showed no difference between the scalp acupuncture group and the Motomed group.

Acupuncture Used as Integrative Medicine

Acupuncture therapy was evaluated in 75 RCTs when it was used in combination with other therapies, including pharmacotherapies or routine care/rehabilitation (A3–A5, A7–A9, A11, A12, A14–A18, A20, A22, A23, A26, A29, A30, A37, A48–A50, A52–A57, A59–A66, A68–A71, A74–A83, A85–A90, A94, A95, A97, A98, A101–A103, A105, A106, A108, A110–A114, A116, A129, A151). The effects of acupuncture tested as an integrative therapy are presented below according to each comparison and outcome. Significant benefit of adding acupuncture to routine care/rehabilitation was proved by meta-analyses of all included outcome measures. The results of meta-analyses are summarised in Table 7.3.

Ashworth Scale or Modified Ashworth Scale

A total of 21 studies (A14, A30, A50, A53, A55, A63, A66, A69, A74, A78, A79, A83, A85, A87, A90, A94, A101, A102, A105, A111,

Table 7.3 Meta-analyses Results: Acupuncture as Integrative Medicine versus Routine Care/Rehabilitation (End of Treatment)

Outcome	No. of Studies	No. of Participants	Effect Size MD/SMD [95% CI]	I^2 (%)	Included Studies
AS or MAS (unspecified)	21	1,572	SMD: −0.48 [−0.58, −0.38] *	0	A14, A30, A50, A53, A55, A63, A66, A69, A74, A78, A79, A83, A85, A87, A90, A94, A101, A102, A105, A111, A151
AS or MAS (upper limb)	8	498	SMD: −0.56 [−0.84, −0.28]*	58	A7, A37, A48, A56, A59, A76, A80, A88
AS or MAS (lower limb)	4	245	SMD: −0.38 [−0.64, −0.13]*	0	A7, A76, A88, A108
FMA (motor)	25	2,013	MD: 11.98 [8.59, 15.36]*	95	A3, A4, A11, A12, A14, A15, A17, A18, A20, A26, A54, A57, A60, A63, A74, A78, A79, A85, A88, A95, A101, A102, A105, A113, A114
FMA (upper limb)	17	1,298	MD: 5.59 [3.98, 7.20]*	60	A5, A8, A9, A14, A16–A18, A50, A56, A59, A66, A75, A80, A88–A90, A112
FMA (lower limb)	15	1,156	MD: 3.11 [2.32, 3.90]*	62	A5, A9, A14, A16, A18, A29, A66, A68, A88, A90, A103, A106, A110, A112, A116
BI	30	2,326	MD: 11.35 [8.62, 14.08]*	84	A3, A5, A16–A18, A26, A37, A49, A53–A55, A57, A60, A63, A68, A69, A74, A78, A79, A81, A82, A85, A90, A95, A101, A102, A111, A113, A114, A116

*Statistically significant.

Abbreviations: AS – Ashworth Scale; BI – Barthel Index; CI – confidence interval; FMA – Fugl-Meyer Assessment; MAS – Modified Ashworth Scale; MD – mean difference; SMD – standardised mean difference.

A151) reported data on AS or MAS (unspecified); meta-analysis showed that the combination of acupuncture and routine care/rehabilitation was more effective than routine care/rehabilitation alone (SMD: –0.48 [–0.58, –0.38], $I^2 = 0\%$).

Eight studies (A7, A37, A48, A56, A59, A76, A80, A88) reported data on AS or MAS (upper limb). Meta-analysis suggested that the combination of acupuncture and routine care/rehabilitation was superior to routine care/rehabilitation alone (SMD: –0.56 [–0.84, –0.28], $I^2 = 58\%$). Meta-analysis of four studies (A7, A76, A88, A108) which reported data on AS or MAS (lower limb) showed that the combination of acupuncture and routine care/rehabilitation was superior to routine care/rehabilitation alone (SMD: –0.38 [–0.64, –0.13], $I^2 = 0\%$).

Fugl-Myer Assessment

Twenty-five studies (A3, A4, A11, A12, A14, A15, A17, A18, A20, A26, A54, A57, A60, A63, A74, A78, A79, A85, A88, A95, A101, A102, A105, A113, A114) reported data on FMA (motor). Meta-analysis of these 25 studies showed that, at the end-of-treatment phase, the combination was more effective than routine care/rehabilitation alone (MD: 11.98 [8.59, 15.36], $I^2 = 95\%$). Only one study (A12) reported data on FMA (motor) at the end of the follow-up phase, showing that there is long-term benefit of combining acupuncture with routine care/rehabilitation (MD: 38.30 [30.09, 46.51]).

Data of FMA (upper limb) was reported by 17 studies (A5, A8, A9, A14, A16–A18, A50, A56, A59, A66, A75, A80, A88–A90, A112). Meta-analysis of these 17 studies suggested the combination of acupuncture and routine case/rehabilitation was more effective than routine case/rehabilitation alone (MD: 5.59 [3.98, 7.20], $I^2 = 60\%$). Fifteen studies (A5, A9, A14, A16, A18, A29, A66, A68, A88, A90, A103, A106, A110, A112, A116) reported data of FMA (lower limb); the combination was more effective than routine care/rehabilitation alone (MD: 3.11 [2.32, 3.90], $I^2 = 62\%$).

Barthel Index

Data of BI was reported by 30 studies (A3, A5, A16–A18, A26, A37, A49, A53–A55, A57, A60, A63, A68, A69, A74, A78, A79, A81, A82, A85, A90, A95, A101, A102, A111, A113, A114, A116), the combination was more effective than routine care/rehabilitation alone (MD: 11.35 [8.62, 14.08], $I^2 = 84\%$).

Assessment Using Grading of Recommendations Assessment, Development and Evaluation

At the conclusion of a consensus process, as described in Chapter 4, it was determined that summary of findings tables should be prepared for the comparison of acupuncture to sham acupuncture, and acupuncture plus rehabilitation compared with rehabilitation alone. In terms of acupuncture compared to sham acupuncture, the evidence of three outcomes from one study was assessed as 'low' to 'moderate' certainty (see Table 7.4); while for the acupuncture used as integrative medicine compared with rehabilitation alone, the evidence of all outcomes was of 'low' certainty, although a significant benefit of adding acupuncture was found (see Table 7.5).

Frequently Reported Acupuncture Points in Meta-analyses Showing Favourable Effects

Among all studies evaluating acupuncture therapy, multiple meta-analyses were conducted for the main outcome measures. The most frequent acupuncture points used in studies from favourable meta-analyses were calculated (Table 7.6). Studies were grouped according to the outcome measures (AS or MAS, FMA, BI) regardless of their comparator (placebo/sham, pharmacotherapy, rehabilitation therapy or add-on comparison).

Among these points, seven points were shown in all frequent point lists of three outcome measures; they were LI4 *Hegu* 合谷, SP6

Table 7.4 GRADE: Acupuncture Compared with Sham Acupuncture for Post-stroke Spasticity

Outcomes	No. of Participants (Studies)	Certainty of the Evidence (GRADE)	Anticipated Absolute Effects: Risk with Sham Acupuncture	Anticipated Absolute Effects: Risk Difference with Acupuncture (95%CI)
MAS	25 (1 RCT)	⊕⊕◯◯ LOW[a,b]	The mean MAS was 3.3 points.	MD **0 points** (0.79 lower to 0.79 higher)
FMA follow up: Mean 12 weeks	238 (1 RCT)	⊕⊕⊕◯ MODERATE[b]	The mean FMA was 56.4 points.	MD **11.48 points higher** (5.68 higher to 17.28 higher)
BI follow up: Mean 12 weeks	238 (1 RCT)	⊕⊕⊕◯ MODERATE[b]	The mean MBI was 61.6 points.	MD **10 points higher** (4.54 higher to 15.46 higher)

The risk in the intervention group (and its 95% confidence interval) is based on the assumed risk in the comparison group and the **relative effect** of the intervention (and its 95% CI).

Abbreviations: BI – Barthel Index; CI – confidence interval; FMA – Fugl-Meyer Assessment; MAS – Modified Ashworth Scale; MBI – Modified Barthel Index; MD – mean difference; RCT – randomised controlled trial.

Notes

[a]Lack of blinding of personnel and assessors.
[b]Small sample size limits certainty of results.

Study References
MAS: A1
FMA: A31
BI: A31

Sanyinjiao 三阴交, TE5 *Waiguan* 外关, LI11 *Quchi* 曲池, ST36 *Zusanli* 足三里, LU5 *Chize* 尺泽 and SP9 *Yinlingquan* 阴陵泉.

Furthermore, *Jin San Zhen* 靳三针 technique and scalp acupuncture were also commonly used in the studies which were included in the pools of meta-analyses showing positive results. The most frequently used points for needling were three points in the temporal area 颞三针 (n = 15), three points on upper limb 上肢挛三针 (n = 5) and three points on lower limb 下肢挛三针 (n = 5).

Table 7.5 GRADE: Acupuncture plus Routine Care/Rehabilitation Compared with Routine Care/Rehabilitation for Post-stroke Spasticity

Outcomes	No. of Participants (Studies) Follow-up	Certainty of the Evidence (GRADE)	Anticipated Absolute Effects	
			Risk with Rehabilitation	Risk Difference with Acupuncture + Rehabilitation (95%CI)
AS or MAS (upper limbs)	498 (8 RCTs)	⊕⊕◯◯ LOW[a,b]	—	SMD **0.56 SD lower** (0.84 lower to 0.28 lower)
AS or MAS (lower limbs)	245 (4 RCTs)	⊕⊕◯◯ LOW[a,c]	—	SMD **0.38 SD lower** (0.64 lower to 0.13 lower)
FMA (motor)	2,013 (25 RCTs)	⊕⊕◯◯ LOW[a,d]	The mean FMA (motor) was **55.59** points.	MD **11.89 points higher** (8.59 higher to 15.36 higher)
FMA (upper limbs)	1,298 (17 RCTs)	⊕⊕◯◯ LOW[a,b]	The mean FMA (upper limbs) was **34.67** points.	MD **5.59 points higher** (3.98 higher to 7.2 higher)
FMA (lower limbs)	986 (15 RCTs)	⊕⊕◯◯ LOW[a,e]	The mean FMA (lower limbs) was **21.77** points.	MD **3.11 points higher** (2.32 higher to 3.9 higher)
BI	2,326 (30 RCTs)	⊕⊕◯◯ LOW[a,d]	The mean BI was **53.57** points.	MD **11.35 points higher** (8.62 higher to 14.08 higher)
Adverse events	147 (2 RCTs)	Two studies reported on adverse events. One study reported six cases of short-term nerve pain or numbness and oedema in both acupuncture and control groups. Another study reported one case of uncomfortable feeling related to haematoma on the head caused by scalp acupuncture		

The risk in the intervention group (and its 95% confidence interval) is based on the assumed risk in the comparison group and the **relative effect** of the intervention (and its 95% CI).

Abbreviations: AS – Ashworth Scale; BI – Barthel Index; CI – confidence interval; FMA – Fugl-Meyer Assessment; MAS – Modified Ashworth Scale; MD – mean difference; RCT – randomised controlled trial; SMD – standardised mean difference.

(Continued)

Table 7.5 (*Continued*)

Notes

[a]Lack of blinding of participants, personnel and assessors.
[b]Moderate statistical heterogeneity.
[c]Small sample size limits certainty of results.
[d]Considerable statistical heterogeneity.
[e]Substantial statistical heterogeneity.

Study References

AS or MAS (upper limbs): A7, A37, A48, A56, A59, A76, A80, A88
AS or MAS (lower limbs): A7, A76, A88, A108
FMA (motor): A3, A4, A11, A12, A14, A15, A17, A18, A20, A26, A54, A57, A60, A63, A74, A78, A79, A85, A88, A95, A101, A102, A105, A113, A114
FMA (upper limbs): A5, A8, A9, A14, A16–A18, A50, A56, A59, A66, A75, A80, A88–A90, A112
FMA (lower limbs): A5, A9, A14, A16, A18, A29, A66, A68, A88, A90, A103, A106, A110, A112, A116
BI: A3, A5, A16–A18, A26, A37, A49, A53–A55, A57, A60, A63, A68, A69, A74, A78, A79, A81, A82, A85, A90, A95, A101, A102, A111, A113, A114, A116
Adverse events: A8, A78

Non-randomised Controlled Trials of Acupuncture

Eleven non-randomised controlled trials involving over 700 participants evaluated the effects of acupuncture (A153–A163). One study (A161) compared acupuncture with routine rehabilitation while the remaining studies investigated the add-on effects of acupuncture to routine rehabilitation or pharmacotherapy. Scalp acupuncture was used in two studies (A155, A163); one study (A157) applied acupuncture on *Jiaji* 夹脊 points and one study (A160) only needled *Jing*-well points. The remaining studies used 39 different acupoints with the most frequently used ones being LI4 *Hegu* 合谷 (*n* = 7), TE5 *Waiguan* 外关 (*n* = 5), SP6 *Sanyinjiao* 三阴交 (*n* = 5), LI10 *Shousanli* 手三里 (*n* = 4), LI11 *Quchi* 曲池 (*n* = 4), SP10 *Xuehai* 血海 (*n* = 4), ST36 *Zusanli* 足三里 (*n* = 4), SI3 *Houxi* 后溪 (*n* = 3), KI6 *Zhaohai* 照海 (*n* = 3) and LI15 *Jianyu* 肩髃 (*n* = 3).

Meta-analysis was only available for the studies investigating the add-on effects of acupuncture. The effects of the main outcomes for acupuncture therapies are presented below.

Table 7.6 Frequently Reported Acupuncture Points in Meta-analyses Showing Favourable Effect

Outcome Measure	No. of Meta-analyses	No. of Studies	Acupuncture Points	Frequency of Use
AS or MAS	4	34	LI4 *Hegu* 合谷	20
			SP6 *Sanyinjiao* 三阴交	19
			TE5 *Waiguan* 外关	15
			LI11 *Quchi* 曲池	14
			ST36 *Zusanli* 足三里	12
			LU5 *Chize* 尺泽	11
			SP10 *Xuehai* 血海	11
			LR3 *Taichong* 太冲	10
			LI10 *Shousanli* 手三里	9
			SP9 *Yinlingquan* 阴陵泉	9
FMA	5	54	SP6 *Sanyinjiao* 三阴交	19
			LI4 *Hegu* 合谷	18
			TE5 *Waiguan* 外关	18
			LI11 *Quchi* 曲池	18
			LU5 *Chize* 尺泽	15
			LR3 *Taichong* 太冲	13
			SP9 *Yinlingquan* 阴陵泉	13
			PC6 *Neiguan* 内关	12
			HT1 *Jiquan* 极泉	12
			ST36 *Zusanli* 足三里	11
BI	1	30	SP6 *Sanyinjiao* 三阴交	16
			LI4 *Hegu* 合谷	14
			LI11 *Quchi* 曲池	12
			SP9 *Yinlingquan* 阴陵泉	11
			TE5 *Waiguan* 外关	10
			LU5 *Chize* 尺泽	10
			LI10 *Shousanli* 手三里	8
			ST36 *Zusanli* 足三里	8
			SP10 *Xuehai* 血海	8
			HT1 *Jiquan* 极泉	8

Abbreviations: AS – Ashworth Scale; BI – Barthel Index; FMA – Fugl-Meyer Assessment; MAS – Modified Ashworth Scale.

Ashworth Scale or Modified Ashworth Scale

Eight studies (A153, A154, A156, A158–A160, A162, A163) reported data on MAS. Meta-analysis of six studies (A153, A154, A158–A160, A163) for MAS (unspecified) (SMD: –0.61 [–0.87, –0.35], I^2 = 38%), and two studies (A156, A162) for MAS (upper limb) (SMD: –0.51 [–0.84, –0.18], I^2 = 0%) both showed a benefit of adding acupuncture to routine therapies.

Fugl-Myer Assessment

Four studies (A153, A155, A158, A159) reported data of FMA (motor) scores. Meta-analysis also showed significant superior effects of the integrated therapy (MD: 8.57 [6.84, 10.29], I^2 = 0%).

Barthel Index

Data on BI was reported in five studies (A153–A156, A159). Significant add-on effects of acupuncture were found (MD: 11.32 [4.84, 17.80], I^2 = 88%).

Non-controlled Clinical Studies of Acupuncture

A total of 33 non-controlled clinical studies of acupuncture for post-stroke spasticity involving 1,518 participants were found from our search (A164, A165, A168–A198). Acupuncture of needling body acupoints was applied in all these studies, with scalp acupuncture also used in four studies (A177, A182, A183, A198).

In total, 112 different points were used in these studies. The most frequently used ones were LI4 *Hegu* 合谷 (*n* = 16), TE5 *Waiguan* 外关 (*n* = 12), LI11 *Quchi* 曲池 (*n* = 11), LI15 *Jianyu* 肩髃 (*n* = 11), ST36 *Zusanli* 足三里 (*n* = 10), SP10 *Xuehai* 血海 (*n* = 9), PC6 *Neiguan* 内关 (*n* = 8), LI10 *Shousanli* 手三里 (*n* = 8), GB34 *Yanglingquan* 阳陵泉 (*n* = 8) and SP9 *Yanglingquan* 三阴交 (*n* = 7).

Safety of Acupuncture

Adverse events were reported in seven RCTs (A8, A37, A57, A58, A72, A78, A97). All CCTs and non-controlled clinical studies did not report information of adverse events. Zhang *et al.* (2011) (A78), reported six cases of short-term nerve pain or numbness and oedema in both acupuncture and control groups; these were considered to be caused by the nerve blocking therapy. Zhuang *et al.* (2009) (A8) reported one case of uncomfortable feeling related to haematoma on the head caused by scalp acupuncture, without any additional management required. The other five studies reported no adverse events in all groups (A37, A57, A58, A72), or no serious adverse event occurred in all groups (A97).

Electroacupuncture

Randomised Controlled Trials of Electroacupuncture

Thirty-nine RCTs (A19, A21, A27, A35, A38, A47, A51, A67, A73, A91–A93, A96, A100, A107, A115, A117–A128, A130–A140) evaluated the effects of electroacupuncture. A total of 2,513 participants were included in these 39 studies. Among them, five studies (A35, A38, A130, A131, A132) compared electroacupuncture with pharmacotherapy, six studies (A47, A51, A118, A135, A137, A140) compared electroacupuncture with routine care/rehabilitation and 31 studies (A19, A21, A27, A47, A51, A67, A73, A91–A93, A96, A100, A107, A115, A117–A128, A133, A134, A136, A138, A139) evaluated the add-on effects of electroacupuncture. Three studies (A47, A51, A118) were three-armed studies which contained three groups: electroacupuncture, routine care/rehabilitation, and the combination of electroacupuncture and routine care/rehabilitation.

Electroacupuncture versus Pharmacotherapy (Baclofen)

Five studies (A35, A38, A130–A132) compared electroacupuncture to baclofen. Three studies (A35, A38, A131) reported data on MAS (unspecified); meta-analysis showed that there was no significant difference between the electroacupuncture and baclofen groups (SMD: –0.10 [–0.41, 0.21], I^2 = 0%). One study (A130) reported data on FMA (upper limb), showing that the electroacupuncture was superior to peraofen for this outcome (MD: 21.84 [17.48, 26.20]). Data of BI was reported by three studies (A35, A38, A130); meta-analysis showed that there was no significant difference between the two therapies (MD: 4.78 [–2.51, 12.08], I^2 = 75%).

Electroacupuncture versus Routine Care/Rehabilitation Alone

Six studies (A47, A51, A118, A135, A137, A140) compared electroacupuncture with routine care/rehabilitation. Meta-analyses on three outcome measures – MAS (unspecified), FMA (motor) and BI – at the end of the treatment phase showed that there was no significant difference between electroacupuncture and routine care/rehabilitation (see Table 7.7). Furthermore, there were results from single studies showing that electroacupuncture was more effective than routine care/rehabilitation for FMA (upper limb) (MD: –1.00 [–1.91, –0.09]) (A47), and FMA (lower limb) (MD: 6.92 [5.98, 7.86]) (A140), at the end-of-treatment phase.

At the end of the follow-up phase, only one study (A135) reported data on FMA (motor) with no significant difference between electroa-

Table 7.7 Meta-analyses Results: Electroacupuncture versus Routine care/ Rehabilitation

Outcome	No. of Studies	No. of Participants	Effect Size [95% CI]	I^2 (%)	Included Studies
MAS (unspecified)	3	200	SMD: 0.38 [–1.38, 2.15]	97	A47, A135, A137
FMA (motor)	3	180	MD: 6.24 [–0.08, 12.55]	62	A51, A135, A137
BI	4	226	MD: –2.56 [–15.41, 10.30]	91	A47, A51, A118, A137

Abbreviations: BI – Barthel Index; CI – confidence interval; FMA – Fugl-Meyer Assessment; MAS – Modified Ashworth Scale; SMD – standardised mean difference.

cupuncture and routine care/rehabilitation being detected (MD: 5.04 [−0.65, 10.73]).

Electroacupuncture Combined with Routine Care/Rehabilitation versus Routine Care/Rehabilitation Alone

A total of 31 studies evaluated the add-on effects of electroacupuncture (A19, A21, A27, A47, A51, A67, A73, A91–A93, A96, A100, A107, A115, A117–A128, A133, A134, A136, A138, A139). Used as an add-on therapy to routine care/rehabilitation, meta-analyses were conducted for the outcomes of MAS (unspecified), MAS (upper limb), MAS (lower limb), FMA (motor), FMA (upper limb), FMA (lower limb), BI or MBI. Results showed that adding electroacupuncture, combined with routine care/rehabilitation, was superior to routine care/rehabilitation alone for MAS (unspecified), MAS (lower limb), FMA (motor), FMA (lower limb) and BI. However, this was not found for the outcomes of MAS (upper limb) and FMA (upper limb). For details, see Table 7.8.

Assessment Using Grading of Recommendations Assessment, Development and Evaluation

Grading of Recommendations Assessment, Development and Evaluation summary of findings tables were prepared for the comparison of electroacupuncture plus routine care/rehabilitation, compared with routine care/rehabilitation alone. The evidence of all outcomes was assessed as 'very low' to 'low' certainty (see Table 7.9).

Frequently Reported Acupuncture Points in Meta-analyses Showing Favourable Effect

Among all studies evaluating electroacupuncture therapy, multiple meta-analyses were found for the main outcome measures. The most frequent herbs used in studies from favourable meta-analyses were calculated (Table 7.10). Studies were grouped according to the outcome measures (AS or MAS, FMA, BI) regardless of their comparator (placebo/sham, pharmacotherapy, rehabilitation therapy, or add-on comparison).

Table 7.8 Meta-analyses Results: Electroacupuncture as Integrative Medicine versus Routine care/Rehabilitation

Outcome	No. of Studies	No. of Participants	Effect Size [95% CI]	I^2 (%)	Included Studies
MAS (unspecified)	10	722	SMD: –0.56 [–1.08, –0.04]*	91	A21, A47, A93, A96, A100, A107, A120, A125, A136, A138
MAS (upper limb)	4	219	SMD: –0.28 [–0.56, 0.01]	10	A92, A122, A124, A133
MAS (lower limb)	3	161	SMD –0.39 [–0.70, –0.08]*	0	A122, A124, A133
FMA (motor)	9	562	MD: 14.17 [8.95, 19.38]*	90	A21, A51, A91, A93, A107, A117, A125, A136, A139
FMA (upper limb)	6	415	MD: 11.54 [–5.80, 28.89]	100	A47, A92, A115, A119, A127, A133
FMA (lower limb)	6	465	MD 4.18 [2.71, 5.65]*	70	A67, A115, A119, A127, A133, A134
BI	14	856	MD: 10.29 [6.64, 13.93]*	87	A21, A47, A51, A67, A91, A93, A107, A115, A118, A120, A121, A125, A127, A139

*Statistically significant.

Abbreviations: BI – Barthel Index; CI – confidence interval; FMA – Fugl-Meyer Assessment; MAS – Modified Ashworth Scale; MD – mean difference; SMD – standardised mean difference.

Among these points, seven were shown in the frequent point lists of three outcome measures; they are LI4 *Hegu* 合谷, TE5 *Waiguan* 外关, LI10 *Shousanli* 手三里, LI11 *Quchi* 曲池, GB34 *Yanglingquan* 阳陵泉, SP6 *Sanyinjiao* 三阴交 and ST36 *Zusanli* 足三里.

Non-randomised Controlled Trials of Electroacupuncture

The add-on effects of electroacupuncture were also evaluated by one non-randomised controlled study (A152). There was no significant

Table 7.9 GRADE: Electroacupuncture plus Rehabilitation versus Rehabilitation for Post-stroke Spasticity

Outcomes	No. of Participants (Studies) Follow-up	Certainty of the Evidence (GRADE)	Anticipated Absolute Effects	
			Risk with Rehabilitation	Risk Difference with Electroacupuncture + Rehabilitation (95%CI)
MAS (upper limbs)	219 (4 RCTs)	⊕⊕◯◯ LOW[a,b]	—	SMD **0.28 SD lower** (0.56 lower to 0.01 higher)
MAS (lower limbs)	161 (3 RCTs)	⊕⊕◯◯ LOW[a,c]	—	SMD **0.39 SD lower** (0.7 lower to 0.08 lower)
FMA (motor)	562 (9 RCTs)	⊕⊕◯◯ LOW[a,d]	The mean FMA was **45.39** points.	MD **14.17 points higher** (8.95 higher to 19.38 higher)
FMA (upper limbs)	415 (6 RCTs)	⊕◯◯◯ VERY LOW[a,d,e]	The mean FMA was **21.88** points.	MD **11.54 points higher** (5.8 lower to 28.89 higher)
FMA (lower limbs)	465 (6 RCTs)	⊕⊕◯◯ LOW[a,f]	The mean FMA was **16.13** points.	MD **4.18 points higher** (2.71 higher to 5.65 higher)
BI	956 (14 RCTs)	⊕⊕◯◯ LOW[a,f]	The mean BI was **56.25** points.	MD **10.29 points higher** (6.64 higher to 13.93 higher)

The risk in the intervention group (and its 95% confidence interval) is based on the assumed risk in the comparison group and the **relative effect** of the intervention (and its 95% CI).

Abbreviations: BI – Barthel Index; CI – confidence interval; FMA – Fugl-Meyer Assessment; MAS – Modified Ashworth Scale; MD – mean difference; RCT – randomised controlled trial; SMD – standardised mean difference.

Notes

[a]Lack of blinding of participants, personnel and assessors.
[b]Small sample size limits certainty of results and 95% CI overlaps no effect.
[c]Small sample size limits certainty of results.
[d]Considerable statistical heterogeneity.
[e]95% CI overlaps no effect.
[f]Substantial statistical heterogeneity.

(*Continued*)

Table 7.9 (*Continued*)

Study References
MAS (upper limbs): A92, A122, A124, A133
MAS (lower limbs): A122, A124, A133
FMA (Motor): A21, A51, A91, A93, A107, A117, A125, A136, A139
FMA (upper limbs): A47, A92, A115, A119, A127, A133
FMA (lower limbs): A67, A115, A119, A127, A133, A134
BI: A21, A47, A51, A67, A91, A93, A107, A115, A118, A120, A121, A125, A127, A139

difference found at the end-of-treatment period for the outcomes of FMA (upper limb) (MD: 1.45 [–0.64, 3.54]) and FMA (lower limb) (MD: 0.89 [–1.17, 2.95]).

Non-controlled Clinical Studies of Electroacupuncture

Two non-controlled clinical studies (A166, A167) reported the effects of electroacupuncture for post-stroke spasticity. A total of 66 participants were involved in these two studies. In these two studies, electroacupuncture was applied on body acupoints with three points being the common ones: LI4 *Hegu* 合谷, LI11 *Quchi* 曲池 and ST36 *Zusanli* 足三里.

Safety of Electroacupuncture

Adverse events were only reported in one RCT (A35). Guan *et al.* (2011) (A35) reported one case of fatigue after electroacupuncture occurred in the intervention group, and 27 cases of adverse events including fatigue, drowsiness, mouth dryness and dizziness caused by medication (baclofen).

Acupressure

Randomised Controlled Trials of Acupressure

Three studies (A141–A143) evaluated the application of pressing acupuncture points for post-stroke spasticity. All three studies (A141–A143) evaluated adding acupressure therapy to routine

Table 7.10 Frequently Reported Acupuncture Points in Meta-analyses Showing Favourable Effect

Outcome Measure	No. of Meta-analyses	No. of Studies	Acupuncture Points	Frequency of Use
AS or MAS	3	13	LI4 *Hegu* 合谷	8
			TE5 *Waiguan* 外关	8
			LI10 *Shousanli* 手三里	7
			LI11 *Quchi* 曲池	7
			LI15 *Jianyu* 肩髃	7
			GB34 *Yanglingquan* 阳陵泉	6
			SP6 *Sanyinjiao* 三阴交	5
			ST36 *Zusanli* 足三里	5
			ST40 *Fenglong* 丰隆	4
			LR3 *Taichong* 太冲	4
FMA	2	16	GB34 *Yanglingquan* 阳陵泉	11
			LI4 *Hegu* 合谷	8
			TE5 *Waiguan* 外关	8
			LI10 *Shousanli* 手三里	7
			LI11 *Quchi* 曲池	6
			ST36 *Zusanli* 足三里	6
			LR3 *Taichong* 太冲	6
			SP6 *Sanyinjiao* 三阴交	5
			SP9 *Yinlingquan* 阴陵泉	4
			LI15 *Jianyu* 肩髃	4
BI	1	14	LI4 *Hegu* 合谷	9
			TE5 *Waiguan* 外关	9
			GB34 *Yanglingquan* 阳陵泉	8
			LI11 *Quchi* 曲池	7
			ST36 *Zusanli* 足三里	7
			LR3 *Taichong* 太冲	7
			LI10 *Shousanli* 手三里	6
			SP6 *Sanyinjiao* 三阴交	5
			GV20 *Baihui* 百会	5
			SP9 *Yinlingquan* 阴陵泉	4

Abbreviations: AS – Ashworth Scale; BI – Barthel Index; FMA – Fugl-Meyer Assessment; MAS – Modified Ashworth Scale.

rehabilitation. Modified Ashworth Scale was reported in two studies, with one study (A141) reporting MAS (unspecified) (MD: –0.80 [–1.30, –0.30]) and another study (A142) reporting MAS (upper limb) (MD: –0.37 [–0.65, –0.09]).

Two studies (A141, A143) reported data on FMA (motor); meta-analysis showed that adding acupressure was superior to routine rehabilitation (MD: 18.98 [1.85, 36.11], I^2 = 92%). Furthermore, BI was only reported by one study (A143) with superior results being found in the acupressure integrative group (MD: 6.15 [0.80, 11.50]). These studies did not report information of adverse events.

Assessment Using Grading of Recommendations Assessment, Development and Evaluation

Grading of Recommendations Assessment, Development and Evaluation summary of finding table shows that the evidence of acupressure combing with rehabilitation compared with rehabilitation for all outcome measures are of 'very low' to 'low' certainty (see Table 7.11).

Moxibustion

Randomised Controlled Trials of Moxibustion

Seven RCTs (A144–A150) evaluated the effects of moxibustion therapy. A total of 529 participants were included in these seven studies. Moxibustion therapy was applied on certain acupuncture points in four studies (A144, A145, A148, A150) and along upper limb meridians in one study (A149). The remaining two studies did not provide this information.

Five studies (A144–A148) compared the combination of moxibustion and routine rehabilitation with routine rehabilitation alone. Another two studies (A149, A150) were three-armed studies which contained three groups: moxibustion, routine care/rehabilitation, and the combination of moxibustion and routine care/rehabilitation.

Table 7.11 GRADE: Acupressure plus Rehabilitation versus Rehabilitation for Post-stroke Spasticity

Outcomes	No. of Participants (Studies) Follow-up	Certainty of the Evidence (GRADE)	Anticipated Absolute Effects	
			Risk with Rehabilitation	Risk Difference with Acupressure + Rehabilitation (95%CI)
MAS (upper limbs)	81 (1 RCT)	⊕⊕◯◯ LOW[a,b]	The mean MAS was **1.6** points.	MD **0.37 points lower** (0.65 lower to 0.09 lower)
FMA (motor)	110 (2 RCTs)	⊕◯◯◯ VERY LOW[a,b,c]	The mean FMA was **39.59** points.	MD **18.98 points higher** (1.85 higher to 36.11 higher)
BI	64 (1 RCT)	⊕⊕◯◯ LOW[a,b]	The mean BI was **37.83** points.	MD **6.15 points higher** (0.8 higher to 11.5 higher)

The risk in the intervention group (and its 95% confidence interval) is based on the assumed risk in the comparison group and the **relative effect** of the intervention (and its 95% CI).

Abbreviations: BI – Barthel Index; CI – confidence interval; FMA – Fugl-Meyer Assessment; MAS – Modified Ashworth Scale; MD – mean difference; RCT – randomised controlled trial.

Notes
[a]Lack of blinding of participants, personnel and assessors.
[b]Small sample size limits certainty of results.
[c]Considerable statistical heterogeneity.

Study References
MAS (upper limbs): A142
FMA (motor): A141, A143
BI: A143

Moxibustion versus Routine Rehabilitation

Two studies (A149, A150) compared moxibustion therapy with routine rehabilitation. Meta-analysis showed that moxibustion therapy was superior to routine rehabilitation for BI (MD: 8.64 [2.88, 14.41], $I^2 = 27\%$).

Moxibustion Used as Integrative Medicine

Seven studies (A144–A150) compared the combination of moxibustion therapy and routine rehabilitation with routine rehabilitation

Table 7.12 Meta-analyses Results: Moxibustion as Integrative Medicine versus Routine Care/Rehabilitation

Outcome	No. of Studies	No. of Participants	Effect Size [95% CI]	I^2 (%)	Included Studies
MAS (unspecified)	2	100	SMD: –0.74 [–1.15, –0.34]*	0	A145, A147
MAS (upper limb)	2	136	SMD: –0.38 [–0.72, –0.04]*	0	A144, A148
FMA (motor)	3	213	MD: 9.32 [7.45, 11.19]*	0	A145–A147
BI	6	356	MD: 14.04 [10.90, 17.18]*	89	A144, A145, A147–A150

*Statistically significant.

Abbreviations: BI – Barthel Index; CI – confidence interval; FMA – Fugl-Meyer Assessment; MAS – Modified Ashworth Scale; MD – mean difference; SMD – standardised mean difference.

alone. Treatment effects are presented for each outcome below. The results of meta-analyses are presented in Table 7.12.

Ashworth Scale or Modified Ashworth Scale

Meta-analyses results showed that adding moxibustion to routine rehabilitation was significantly more effective than routine rehabilitation alone for MAS (unspecified) (SMD: –0.74 [–1.15, –0.34], $I^2 = 0\%$) (A145, A147) and MAS (upper limb) (SMD: –0.38 [–0.72, –0.04], $I^2 = 0\%$) (A144, A148).

Fugl-Meyer Assessment

Three studies (A145–A147) reported data on FMA (motor). The meta-analysis result is in favour of the combination of moxibustion therapy and routine rehabilitation (MD: 9.32 [7.45, 11.19], $I^2 = 0\%$). One study (A148) reported data on FMA (upper limb); the combination is more effective than routine rehabilitation (MD 13.51 [12.72, 14.30]). One study (A148) reported data on a simplified version of FMA (lower limb), with the combination being superior to routine rehabilitation alone (MD: 2.97 [2.61, 3.33]).

Barthel Index

Six studies (A144, A145, A147–A150) reported data on BI. It was found that adding moxibustion to routine rehabilitation is more effective than routine rehabilitation alone (MD: 14.04 [10.90, 17.18], I^2 = 89%). A further two studies (A149, A150) also reported data on BI at the end of the follow-up phase, showing a significantly positive result (MD: 14.94 [9.08, 20.81], I^2 = 44%). These studies did not report information of adverse events.

Assessment Using Grading of Recommendations Assessment, Development and Evaluation

In Grading of Recommendations Assessment, Development and Evaluation the summary of findings table shows that the evidence of moxibustion combined with rehabilitation, compared with rehabilitation alone, for all outcome measures are of 'low' certainty (see Table 7.13).

Acupuncture plus Moxibustion

Randomised Controlled Trials of Acupuncture plus Moxibustion

Three studies (A24, A99, A109) assessed the add-on effects of acupuncture plus moxibustion. All three studies used the combination of acupuncture and moxibustion, in addition to routine care/rehabilitation. Of these three studies, two studies (A24, A99) applied moxibustion on top of acupuncture needles, and one study (A109) separated acupuncture and moxibustion on different points. It was stated that the method of needling points located on antagonistic muscles and applying moxibustion on spastic muscles of the paralysed extremity is beneficial for reducing spasticity (A109).

Table 7.13 GRADE: Moxibustion plus Rehabilitation versus Rehabilitation for Post-stroke Spasticity

Outcomes	No. of Participants (Studies) Follow-up	Certainty of the Evidence (GRADE)	Anticipated Absolute Effects: Risk with Rehabilitation	Anticipated Absolute Effects: Risk Difference with Moxibustion + Rehabilitation (95%CI)
MAS (upper limbs)	136 (2 RCTs)	⊕⊕◯◯ LOW[a,b]	—	SMD **0.38 SD lower** (0.72 lower to 0.04 lower)
FMA motor	213 (3 RCTs)	⊕⊕◯◯ LOW[a,b]	The mean FMA was **54.18** points.	MD **9.32 points higher** (7.45 higher to 11.19 higher)
FMA (upper limbs)	68 (1 RCT)	⊕⊕◯◯ LOW[a,b]	The mean FMA was **23.13** points.	MD **13.51 points higher** (12.72 higher to 14.3 higher)
FMA (lower limbs)	68 (1 RCT)	⊕⊕◯◯ LOW[a,b]	The mean FMA (lower limbs) was **22.34** points.	MD **2.97 points higher** (2.61 higher to 3.33 higher)
BI	356 (6 RCTs)	⊕⊕◯◯ LOW[a,c]	The mean BI was **53.71** points.	MD **14.04 points higher** (10.9 higher to 17.18 higher)

The risk in the intervention group (and its 95% confidence interval) is based on the assumed risk in the comparison group and the **relative effect** of the intervention (and its 95% CI).

Abbreviations: AS – Ashworth Scale; BI – Barthel Index; CI – confidence interval; FMA – Fugl-Meyer Assessment; MAS – Modified Ashworth Scale; MD – mean difference; RCT – randomised controlled trial; SMD – standardised mean difference.

Notes

[a]Lack of blinding of participants, personnel and assessors.

[b]Small sample size limits certainty of results.

[c]Considerable statistical heterogeneity.

Study References

AS or MAS (upper limbs): A144, A148

FMA (motor): A145, A146, A147

FMA (upper limbs): A148

FMA (lower limbs): A148

BI: A144, A145, A147–A150

One study (A99) reported data on AS (unspecified), but with incorrect scale (68.53 versus 32.12); therefore this was not included in our analysis. One study (A109) reported data on MAS (upper limb); it was found that adding the combination of acupuncture and moxibustion to routine care/rehabilitation achieved superior effects (MD: –0.75 [–1.43, –0.07]).

For other outcome measures, meta-analysis of two studies (A24, A99) showed that adding acupuncture and moxibustion was beneficial for BI (MD: 17.28 [6.52, 28.05], I^2 = 89%), and results of single studies showed that this method also improved the outcomes. One study (A99) reported data on FMA (motor) (MD: 14.11 [11.36, 16.86]), and another study (A24) reported FMA (lower limb) (MD: 8.05 [7.18, 8.92]). Both achieved significant add-on effects but meta-analysis was not available. There was no information of adverse events reported in the included study.

Evidence for Acupuncture and Related Therapies Commonly Used in Clinical Practice

Acupuncture therapies are commonly used to manage post-stroke spasticity in clinical trials, and some of them are also recommended in current guidelines and textbooks (see Chapter 2 for more details). Based on the evidence collected from clinical research, body acupuncture or electroacupuncture are the most popular treatments among the included clinical trials. Other acupuncture-related therapies, including acupressure and moxibustion, have also been evaluated by a small number of studies. In addition, some recently developed special acupuncture techniques, including scalp acupuncture, have been repeatedly utilised in combination with other body acupuncture techniques in clinical trials, although these have not been recommended in the literature (Chapter 2). The evidence of these therapies may enrich the existing clinical practice.

Warm needling, the method of applying moxibustion cones on top of acupuncture needles, has been recommended by contemporary literature (Chapter 2). Although the term 'warm needling'

温针 has not been shown in the included clinical studies, the technique of combining acupuncture and moxibustion has been investigated and proved beneficial for post-stroke spasticity. It is interesting to note that acupuncture and moxibustion can also be applied separately, with needling points located on antagonistic muscles and applying moxibustion on spastic muscles of the paralysed extremity.

Pooling the clinical studies included in meta-analyses showed positive results; two lists of frequently used acupuncture points, according to different outcome measures, were generated (Table 7.6, Table 7.10). The points included in these lists were partially consistent with those that have been recommended in Chapter 2. It is worth noting that some acupuncture points which may have contributed to clinical effects are not included in the recommendations of Chapter 2; they are SP6 *Sanyinjiao* 三阴交, ST36 *Zusanli* 足三里, SP9 *Yinlingquan* 阴陵泉 and HT1 *Jiquan* 极泉.

Summary of Acupuncture and Related Therapies Clinical Evidence

Acupuncture therapies are the most common Chinese medicine treatments used in clinical practice for treating post-stroke spasticity. Our evaluation of clinical studies found that acupuncture therapies could improve clinically relevant outcomes of patients with post-stroke spasticity.

A sufficient number of clinical studies were included in our evaluation; therefore it is feasible to summarise the efficacy of acupuncture-related therapies, as well as extract information related to clinical practice such as Chinese medicine syndromes and acupuncture points. The most common syndrome seen in clinical studies was 'Liver *yang* uprising, Wind and Phlegm blocking the meridians, with *qi* deficiency and Blood stasis'. Efficacy and points used in each category of acupuncture therapies were analysed separately.

Firstly, there has been promising evidence from clinical studies supporting the use of needling acupuncture. In the included studies, acupuncture had been compared to placebo/sham, pharmacotherapy, or routine care/rehabilitation, or been used as an add-on therapy. Outcome measures included in our analyses are mainly focusing on the severity of spasticity (AS or MAS), motor function (FMA) and patients' daily activities (BI).

When acupuncture was used alone, it was reported by a large-scale study (n = 138) that needling Wang's *Jiaji* points 王氏挟脊穴 with *Deqi* 得气 sensation achieved better long-term effects than sham acupuncture for improving patients' motor function (FMA). However, meta-analysis confirming the superior effects of acupuncture over sham/placebo was not feasible due to the very small number of eligible studies.

Compared to pharmacotherapy or routine care/rehabilitation, meta-analyses results suggest that acupuncture achieved greater effects than pharmacotherapy alone for AS or MAS (upper limb) and FMA (upper limb), and acupuncture achieved greater effects than routine care/rehabilitation alone for FMA (motor). As for other outcomes, there was no significant difference between acupuncture and the comparator, either pharmacotherapy or routine care/rehabilitation.

When acupuncture was used as an add-on therapy, meta-analyses results support the use of acupuncture for all outcomes. Evidence showed that adding acupuncture could significantly improve the treatment effects of routine care/rehabilitation for outcome measures of AS or MAS (unspecified), AS or MAS (upper limb), AS or MAS (lower limb), FMA (motor), FMA (upper limb), FMA (lower limb) and BI.

The certainty of evidence of acupuncture compared to placebo and acupuncture being used as integrative medicine compared to routine care/rehabilitation alone have been assessed using the GRADE approach. Most of these evidences were assessed as 'low' certainty, except for the results of FMA and MBI of acupuncture versus placebo which was of 'moderate' certainty. This reflects the fact that the majority of included RCTs contained methodological weaknesses.

By summarising the studies which were included in the meta-analyses with positive results, it was found that similar points may have contributed to the positive effects of three main outcome measures. Seven acupuncture points were shown in all lists; they are LI4

Hegu 合谷, SP6 *Sanyinjiao* 三阴交, TE5 *Waiguan* 外关, LI11 *Quchi* 曲池, ST36 *Zusanli* 足三里, LU5 *Chize* 尺泽 and SP9 *Yinlingquan* 阴陵泉. These may be considered as effective points for clinical practice of acupuncture for post-stroke spasticity. The combination of needling three points on the temporal area (颞三针), three points on upper limb (上肢挛三针) and three points on lower limb (下肢挛三针) may also have contributed to the positive effects brought by meta-analyses. Furthermore, acupuncture can be considered as a safe treatment for post-stroke spasticity. Of all acupuncture studies included in our evaluation, adverse events caused by acupuncture were very rare (only one case was reported) and it did not require any additional medical management.

Electroacupuncture has also been evaluated by clinical studies. Comparing electroacupuncture with routine care/rehabilitation, meta-analyses results showed that there was no significant difference between these therapies for MAS (unspecified), FMA (motor) and BI. When used as an add-on therapy, meta-analyses indicated that adding electroacupuncture could significantly improve the treatment effects in terms of MAS (unspecified), MAS (lower limb), FMA (motor), FMA (lower limb) and BI. Nevertheless, the certainty of evidence for electroacupuncture being used as integrative medicine was assessed using the GRADE approach, with all results being of 'low' certainty.

The electroacupuncture points that may have contributed to the positive effects of meta-analyses for three main outcome measures were similar to those that had been used for acupuncture. There were seven points shown in all lists; they are LI4 *Hegu* 合谷, TE5 *Waiguan* 外关, LI10 *Shousanli* 手三里, LI11 *Quchi* 曲池, GB34 *Yanglingquan* 阳陵泉, SP6 *Sanyinjiao* 三阴交 and ST36 *Zusanli* 足三里. These may be considered as effective points for clinical practice of electroacupuncture for post-stroke spasticity.

Moreover, acupressure and moxibustion have also been evaluated by clinical research and been proved effective and safe when used as add-on therapies for the management of post-stroke spasticity. However, the evidence of acupressure and moxibustion as add-on therapies was assessed as 'low' or 'very low' certainty for all outcomes, using the GRADE approach.

In summary, acupuncture and related therapies show promising treatment effects to improve clinical outcomes for post-stroke spasticity. It is worth noting that there is more evidence for acupuncture and electroacupuncture than other therapies for patients with spasticity. Since the studies included in positive meta-analyses of acupuncture and electroacupuncture share similar frequently used points, the acupuncture points of LI4 *Hegu* 合谷, TE5 *Waiguan* 外关, LI11 *Quchi* 曲池 and ST36 *Zusanli* 足三里 can be considered as the basis of acupuncture prescription for the management of post-stroke spasticity. However, due to the methodological weakness of clinical studies including lack of blinding of participants, inappropriate methods of sequence generation and allocation concealment, these results should be interpreted with caution. In particular, when acupuncture therapies were used as add-on therapy to routine care/rehabilitation, none of the studies applied a sham/placebo control. Therefore, potential placebo effects caused by an additional therapy cannot be ruled out from the significant add-on effects detected by our meta-analyses.

References

1. Park SW, Yi SH, Lee JA, *et al.* (2014) Acupuncture for the treatment of spasticity after stroke: A meta-analysis of randomized controlled trials. *J Altern Complement Med* **20(9):** 672–682.
2. Lim SM, Yoo J, Lee E, *et al.* (2015) Acupuncture for spasticity after stroke: A systematic review and meta-analysis of randomized controlled trials. *Evid Based Complement Alternat Med* **2015**: 870398.

References to Included Clinical Studies

Study ID	References
A1	Fink M, Rollnic JD, Bijak M, *et al.* (2004) Needle Acupuncture in chronic poststroke leg spasticity. *Arch Phys Med Rehabil* **85:** 667–672.
A2	Hussain T, Mohammad H. (2013) The effect of transcutaneous electrical nerve stimulation (TENS) combined with Bobath on post stroke spasticity: A randomized controlled study. *Neurol Sci* **333:** e560.

(*Continued*)

Study ID	References
A3	郎建英, 庄礼兴, 贾超, 贺君, 周昭辉, 韩德雄, 周丹, 蔡小敏, 陈子平. (2011) '靳三针'结合康复疗法治疗缺血性中风痉挛性偏瘫的临床疗效观察. 广州中医药大学学报 **28(4):** 369–373.
A4	陆彦青, 杨海涛, 庄礼兴, 刘悦. (2013) '靳三针'联合康复训练治疗中风后痉挛性偏瘫患者 40 例临床观察. 中医杂志 **54(12):** 1034–1037.
A5	郎建英, 庄礼兴, 贺君, 贾超, 周昭辉, 柯丽萍. (2013) '靳三针'疗法治疗缺血性中风后痉挛性偏瘫随机对照研究. 上海针灸杂志 **32(6):** 440–443.
A6	贺君, 庄礼兴, 郎建英, 韩为, 李丽霞, 徐世芬, 包永欣. (2011) 靳三针对卒中后痉挛性瘫痪患者神经功能缺损和日常生活能力的影响——多中心随机对照研. 新中医 **43(6):** 99–101.
A7	沈巍, 孙曌, 庄礼兴. (2010) 靳三针结合康复治疗缺血性脑卒中后痉挛瘫的临床研究. 辽宁中医杂志 **37(11):** 2228–2230.
A8	庄礼兴, 徐世芬, 庄珣. (2009) 靳三针疗法配合功能训练对脑卒中偏瘫患者上肢功能的影响(英文). *World J Acupunct Moxibustion* **19(4):** 1–6.
A9	庄珣, 贾超, 贺君, 韩德雄, 姜桂美, 庄礼兴. (2010) 靳三针疗法为主治疗脑梗塞偏瘫 40 例. 现代中医药 **30(1):** 52–54.
A10	郎建英, 庄礼兴, 贾超, 贺君, 周昭辉, 柯丽萍, 周丹, 蔡小敏, 陈子平. (2011) 靳三针疗法治疗缺血性中风后痉挛性偏瘫临床观察. 新中医 **43(11):** 93–95.
A11	杨海涛, 庄礼兴, 刘悦. (2013) 靳三针治疗中风后痉挛性偏瘫临床研究及其对康复训练的影响. 辽宁中医杂志 **40(11):** 2349–2351.
A12	杨海涛. (2013) 颞三针配合挛三针治疗中风后痉挛性偏瘫的临床研究 (Thesis). 广州中医药大学.
A13	黄维媚. (2009) 靳三针治疗缺血性中风后偏瘫的临床研究 (Thesis). 广州中医药大学.
A14	占大权. (2009) 靳三针配合作业疗法治疗中风后硬瘫的临床疗效观察 (Thesis). 广州中医药大学.
A15	周昭辉. (2010) 靳三针疗法治疗缺血性中风偏瘫的临床研究 (Thesis). 广州中医药大学.
A16	贾超. (2009) 靳三针疗法治疗脑梗塞偏瘫的规范化研究 (Thesis). 广州中医药大学.
A17	韩德雄. (2010) 靳三针疗法结合康复训练治疗缺血性卒中偏瘫的疗效研究 (Thesis). 广州中医药大学.

(*Continued*)

(*Continued*)

Study ID	References
A18	郎建英. (2011) 靳三针疗法结合康复训练治疗缺血性中风后痉挛性偏瘫的疗效研究 (Thesis). 广州中医药大学.
A19	卢君艳, 屠文展, 张丹迎, 谢文霞, 李劲民, 蒋松鹤. (2010) 不同穴位针刺结合康复训练对偏瘫患者肌痉挛的影响. 中国针灸 **30(7):** 542–546.
A20	佟帅, 苏李, 吕海波, 刘建桥. (2013) 关键点针刺法配合康复治疗脑梗死后痉挛期偏瘫疗效观察. 中国针灸 **33(5):** 399–402.
A21	郭京伟. (2003) 针刺疗法在脑卒中早期康复中的应用研究 (Thesis). 北京中医药大学.
A22	杨娟. (2011) 通督调神针刺法治疗缺血性中风偏瘫的临床研究 (Thesis). 广州中医药大学.
A23	周春宇, 蒲荣, 郑文振, 何兴辉. (2013) 针刺穴位治疗脑卒中痉挛性偏瘫的效果观察. 中国现代药物应用 **7(14):** 44–45.
A24	石新燕, 李小生. (2013) 针灸结合康复治疗对脑卒中偏瘫患者治疗效果的研究. 陕西中医 **34(7):** 877–878.
A25	贾雪梅, 周宇超, 黄亦璇. (2011) 针灸治疗卒中后痉挛性瘫痪状态的临床研究. 临床医学工程 **18(5):** 736–737.
A26	胡非非. (2011) 针康法结合神经干细胞移植对脑梗死患者运动功能恢复的影响 (Thesis). 黑龙江中医药大学.
A27	卢健敏. (2003) 针刺配合康复训练治疗中风后足下垂的临床观察 (Thesis). 福建中医学院.
A28	余芳菲, 郑侠海, 曾科学, 许能贵. (2013) 调任通督针刺法治疗缺血性中风后痉挛性偏瘫 32 例临床观察. 云南中医中药杂志 **34(7):** 50–52.
A29	杨丹, 姜美玉, 杨孝芳, 葛耘, 曾贤, 刘明辉. (2014) 针刺跷脉穴配合康复治疗中风后足内翻疗效观察. 上海针灸杂志 **33(4):** 299–302.
A30	赵力生, 王建文, 杨江霞. (2013) 针刺三阳穴结合抗痉挛牵张技术治疗脑卒中偏瘫患者腕关节痉挛 40 例疗效观察. 甘肃中医学院学报 **30(3):** 67–69.
A31	Li HQ, Liu HL, Liu CZ, *et al.* (2013) Effect of *Deqi* during the study of needling Wang's *Jiaji* acupoints treating spasticity after stroke. *Evid Based Complement Alternat Med* 1–8.
A32	毕颖, 候群, 李丽萍, 邵晓梅, 宣丽华. (2011) 粗针平刺身柱穴配合体针治疗中风后痉挛性瘫痪的临床研究. 中华中医药杂志 **26(6):** 1443–1445.
A33	毕颖, 李丽萍, 冯辉, 宣丽华, 张海峰. (2009) 粗针治疗卒中偏瘫痉挛状态的临床研究. 中华中医药学刊 **27(10):** 2167–2169.

(*Continued*)

(*Continued*)

Study ID	References
A34	韩淑凯. (2015) 经筋排刺法结合皮肤针对脑卒中后上肢偏瘫患者痉挛状态的影响: 多中心随机照研究. *World J Acupunct Moxibustion* **21(7):** 13–18.
A35	关莹, 张立, 邢艳丽, 唐强. (2011) 针康法对脑卒中后痉挛状态的影响. 中国康复理论与实践 **17(4):** 325–327.
A36	张志强. (2007) 针刺夹脊穴治疗卒中后痉挛性瘫痪的临床研究 (Thesis). 广州中医药大学.
A37	王家颖. (2014) 恢刺结合康复训练对脑卒中后上肢偏瘫痉挛状态和生活质量影响的临床研究 (Thesis). 南京中医药大学.
A38	刘俊. (2008) 电针治疗中风后痉挛状态的临床研究 (Thesis). 哈尔滨: 黑龙江省中医研究院.
A39	赵晓峰, 李平. (2005)'补缓泻急'针刺法治疗中风性肌痉挛疗效观察. 上海针灸杂志 **24(10):** 13–14.
A40	史文红, 李雪萍, 王伟, 周俊, 陈安亮, 程凯. (2010) 康复治疗对脑卒中患者腓肠肌表面肌电信号的影响. 中国康复 **25(2):** 103–105.
A41	司世雷. (2014) 平衡针灸法治疗卒中后痉挛性偏瘫 60 例临床观察. 中医临床研究 **6(10):** 37–38, 41.
A42	张红岩, 李佩芳. (2012) 通督调神针刺法治疗缺血性脑卒中后痉挛性瘫痪的临床观察. 四川中医 **30(9):** 123–125.
A43	杜琳, 刘娜, 廖贺, 郭麒竹, 梁湘钰, 赵晋昕, 杨文丽, 魏良燕, 蔡承穆, 金真希. (2014) 温通阴跷法治疗中风足内翻疗效观察. 中华中医药杂志 **29(4):** 1189–1191.
A44	刘婧, 鲍春龄, 张桂波, 焦志华, 东贵荣. (2014) 阴阳调衡透刺法对中风后痉挛瘫患者行走功能重建的影响. 上海针灸杂志 **33(1):** 7–10.
A45	武平, 梁繁荣, 杨玲, 罗伦, 李安宏. (2009) 针刺对脑卒中后偏瘫肢体痉挛患者神经功能缺损的影响. 针灸临床杂志 **25(6):** 8–10.
A46	徐亚莉, 金建军. (2010) 针刺疗法对偏瘫上肢肌痉挛正中神经 f 波波幅及疗效的影响. 中国自然医学杂志 **12(1):** 44–46.
A47	蔡华安, 廖若夷, 张雅珍, 黄文韬, 欧阳文湘, 成国华. (2011) 神经发育促进技术合针刺治疗脑卒中痉挛期 30 例. 湖南中医杂志 **27(4):** 65–66.
A48	陈健安, 余康潮, 钟正, 郑禹, 曲姗姗, 黄泳. (2015) 针刺董氏奇穴和康复训练对脑卒中后上肢痉挛性偏瘫患者的效果. 中国康复理论与实践 **21(3):** 330–333.

(*Continued*)

(*Continued*)

Study ID	References
A49	武平, 梁繁荣, 胡卡明, 田卫卫, 袁秀丽, 黄银兰. (2009) 针刺复合易化技术治疗脑卒中后偏瘫肢体痉挛的临床研究—附: 160 例病例报告. 成都中医药大学学报 **32(1):** 11–13.
A50	曹秦宁, 乔鸿飞. (2012) 针刺拮抗肌联合康复治疗对急性脑卒中偏瘫痉挛状态的影响. 医学美学美容: 中旬刊 **33(11):** 1530–1532.
A51	冉小青, 吴松, 叶丹屏, 闵洁. (2013) 针刺结合康复训练对中风痉挛性偏瘫患者肢体功能及下肢血流的影响. 湖北中医杂志 **35(10):** 20–21.
A52	武平, 梁繁荣, 李瑛, 金荣疆, 胡卡明, 田卫卫, 罗伦, 袁秀丽. (2010) 针刺配合康复训练治疗脑卒中后偏瘫肢体痉挛的疗效评价研究. 世界针灸杂志 (英文版) **20(2):** 1–7.
A53	张瑛, 陈万票, 王晨瑶, 谢腾, 王淼, 夏燕军, 王雅莉. (2014) 针灸解痉调气法结合康复治疗脑卒中痉挛期患者临床评价. 浙江中西医结合杂志 **24(4):** 290–292.
A54	朱冬梅. (2003) 针康法治疗急性脑梗死运动功能障碍的临床观察 (Thesis). 黑龙江中医药大学.
A55	罗清平. (2007) 针刺结合现代康复治疗中风后痉挛性瘫的临床观察 (Thesis). 湖南中医学院.
A56	金成旭. (2010) 针刺结合康复治疗中风偏瘫上肢痉挛状态的临床研究 (Thesis). 黑龙江省中医研究院.
A57	武娜. (2014) 腹针结合康复训练治疗缺血性中风偏瘫痉挛状态的疗效研究 (Thesis). 山西中医学院.
A58	张自茂. (2006) 针刺治疗脑卒中后上肢痉挛的临床疗效研究 (Thesis). 广州医学院.
A59	肖清宁. (2011) 25 例针刺配合康复训练治疗脑卒中后上肢痉挛效果评价. 亚太传统医药 **7(8):** 62–63.
A60	张为民, 郑鹏. (2011) 拮抗肌侧取穴针刺结合现代康复训练疗法治疗中风后痉挛. 世界中西医结合杂志 **6(4):** 291–293, 301.
A61	胡东霞, 彭慧. (2013) 康复训练结合头针对脑梗死后肢体痉挛患者肌张力及神经功能的影响. 实用临床医学 **14(7):** 25–26, 29.
A62	塔长峰, 吴定奇, 马腾飞. (2011) 祛瘀生新针法配合康复训练治疗高血压基底节区脑出血术后痉挛性瘫痪的临床观察. 湖南中医药大学学报 **31(6):** 54–55.

(*Continued*)

(***Continued***)

Study ID	References
A63	何正超, 陈冬, 王明伟, 周林, 汪海东. (2009) 头针结合 Bobath 治疗脑卒中后痉挛的疗效分析. 老年医学与保健 **15(3):** 184–185.
A64	郭严. (2015) 头针结合康复训练治疗中风痉挛性瘫痪55例. 河南中医 **(2):** 278–280.
A65	夏毅. (2011) 头针结合康复训练治疗中风痉挛性瘫痪的疗效观察. 光明中医 **26(8):** 1640–1641.
A66	何小花, 张丽君, 李惠淑, 赵雪岩, 葛文艳, 吕红梅. (2011) 头针配合抗痉挛手法治疗脑卒中后偏瘫痉挛状态的疗效分析. 中国伤残医学 **16(9):** 55–57.
A67	王魁, 刘经星, 杨翊, 徐明权, 杨清. (2013) 透刺配合康复训练对脑卒中后患侧下肢功能的影响. 上海针灸杂志 **32(7):** 539–541.
A68	尹正录, 孟兆祥, 薛永骥, 陈波. (2013) 针刺对脑卒中偏瘫患者踝内翻的疗效观察. 中国康复理论与实践 **19(12):** 1163–1166.
A69	李红星, 罗利敏, 刘东坡, 周红芳. (2011) 针刺拮抗肌侧腧穴治疗中风后肢体痉挛临床观察. 上海针灸杂志 **30(4):** 252–253.
A70	钟素华, 韦继流, 陆丽梅. (2014) 针刺拮抗肌相应穴位结合 Bobath 疗法治疗偏瘫痉挛状态 120 例临床观察. 中国卫生产业 **11(4):** 180–181.
A71	蒋鹏, 郑祖艳. (2013) 针刺拮抗肌相应穴位结合 Bobath 疗法治疗偏瘫痉挛状态的临床观察. 针灸临床杂志 **29(1):** 18–20.
A72	哈静, 冶尕西, 贾红云, 黄银兰, 万明雨, 曹丽翠, 王磊. (2013) 针刺拮抗肌组腧穴治疗脑卒中后偏瘫肢体痉挛的临床研究. 时珍国医国药 **24(2):** 416–418.
A73	任亚锋. (2008) 针刺结合康复疗法治疗卒中后痉挛的临床研究. 光明中医 **6(23):** 426–428.
A74	曾海辉, 伍少玲, 黄利荣, 马超, 金冬梅. (2005) 针刺结合康复训练改善脑卒中后肌肉痉挛的临床研究. 中国康复医学杂志 **20(11):** 846–847.
A75	倪欢欢, 胡永善, 崔晓, 吴毅, 黄德权, 瞿佩育, 汪军, 吴佶, 史骏超. (2011) 针刺结合康复训练治疗脑卒中后上肢痉挛 20 例临床观察. 新中医 **43(1):** 99–101.
A76	杨晓莲, 朱振莉, 孟庆丽, 方亚群. (2008) 针刺结合康复训练治疗脑卒中后肢体痉挛的临床观察. 中华物理医学与康复杂志 **30(7):** 441–442.
A77	张宁. (2013) 针刺结合强迫疗法治疗脑卒中后上肢运动功能障碍的临床研究. 针灸临床杂志 **29(12):** 12–14.

(*Continued*)

(Continued)

Study ID	References
A78	张宝霞, 张金生, 马松鹤. (2011) 针刺结合神经干阻滞治疗中风痉挛性偏瘫的临床观察. 新中医 **(3):** 97–99.
A79	陈新, 陈越峰, 茅敏, 牟欣, 饶萍, 白杨. (2010) 针刺结合现代康复技术治疗中风偏瘫痉挛状态的临床研究. 成都中医药大学学报 **4(15):** 27–29.
A80	王正田. (2013) 针刺结合现代康复疗法对卒中后上肢痉挛状态的疗效观察. 湖南中医药大学学报 **33(4):** 94–95.
A81	王常鸿. (2013) 针刺结合穴位按摩治疗中风后手指屈曲拘挛的临床价值对照研究. 中国民康医学 **25(4):** 55–56.
A82	王英. (2012) 针刺结合运动疗法治疗卒中后足内翻 60 例疗效观察. 河北中医 **34(3):** 412–413.
A83	徐飞, 谢昕, 汪敏娜, 张倩. (2015) 针刺联合康复训练治疗脑梗死后肢体痉挛的疗效观察. 中国实用医药 **10(9):** 284–285.
A84	张瑛, 朱晨曦, 谢腾, 王淼, 夏燕军. (2010) 针刺解痉调气法治疗脑卒中痉挛期患者疗效观察. 中华全科医学 **8(9):** 1155–1156.
A85	金曦. (2012) 针刺联合现代康复训练对中风后肢体痉挛疗效观察. 中国医药指南 **10(10):** 263–264.
A86	王利春, 刘海燕, 王庆海. (2011) 针刺内关联合 Bobath 康复训练治疗脑卒中后全手肌痉挛对照研究. 中国中医药信息杂志 **18(6):** 82–83.
A87	李怡, 李雨峰, 潘福琼, 常有军, 徐嘉, 肖宗欣, 杨玉龙, 陈杰, 赵冠兰. (2008) 针刺配合 Bobath 疗法改善脑卒中后肢体痉挛状态的临床研究. 中国康复理论与实践 **14(11):** 1063–1064.
A88	严伟, 霍文璟, 殷建权. (2003) 针刺配合康复训练缓解中风偏瘫痉挛. 心血管康复医学杂志 **12(4):** 370–371.
A89	倪欢欢, 崔晓, 胡永善, 吴毅, 黄德权, 瞿佩育, 汪军, 吴佶, 史骏超. (2012) 针刺配合康复训练治疗脑卒中后上肢痉挛疗效观察. 上海针灸杂志 **31(11):** 789–791.
A90	邱林, 刘艳春. (2014) 针刺配合康复训练治疗中风后痉挛性偏瘫疗效观察. 河南中医 **51(7):** 1827–1828.
A91	吴威. (2011) 针刺配合康复训练治疗中风偏瘫侧足内翻疗效观察. 上海针灸杂志 **30(5):** 321–323.
A92	郭晋斌, 杨路庭, 路怀忠. (2015) 针刺为主治疗脑梗死后上肢功能障碍临床观察. 光明中医 **30(1):** 90–91.
A93	钟长明, 林洪茂, 刘庆芳, 金红阳. (2001) 针刺与肌张力平衡促通法对中风偏瘫患者早期康复的作用. 中国康复医学杂志 **(3):** 52–54.

(*Continued*)

(*Continued*)

Study ID	References
A94	李志钢, 闫琪, 宋兆炎. (2014) 针刺治疗脑卒中致痉挛疗效观察. 按摩与康复医学 **5(5):** 65–66.
A95	屈春艳. (2014) 针刺治疗在中风痉挛性偏瘫中的疗效观察. 中医临床研究 **6(17):** 18–19.
A96	邢雪梅, 杨波, 李方, 吴疆, 王妍萍. (2015) 针灸联合康复训练治疗缺血性中风后痉挛性偏瘫 30 例. 辽宁中医杂志 **42(3):** 595–597.
A97	薛青理. (2014) 针灸联合西药治疗中风恢复期随机平行对照研究. 实用中医内科杂志 **27(9):** 125–126.
A98	冯绪刚, 赵思宇, 于璐. (2012) 针灸配合康复训练治疗脑卒中痉挛瘫痪的临床观察. 当代医学 **18(27):** 83–84.
A99	吴红新. (2013) 针灸治疗脑卒中后痉挛性偏瘫临床研究. 中医学报 **28(11):** 1761–1762.
A100	王桂华, 关莹, 马晓东. (2007) 针药结合治疗脑卒中后肌张力增高的临床观察. 中医药学报 **35(4):** 41–42.
A101	张治方. (2011) 中医康复与现代康复技术共同治疗卒中后痉挛性偏瘫的研究. 社区中医药 **13(33):** 142–143.
A102	宋俊杰. (2012) 中风后肢体痉挛诊疗技术的研究 (Thesis). 长春中医药大学.
A103	陈艳琴. (2009) 针灸配合康复治疗对中风偏瘫后足下垂疗效的表面肌电研究 (Thesis). 南京中医药大学.
A104	Kazemi, AH. (2010) 针刺治疗中风后下肢痉挛状态的临床观察 (Thesis). 北京中医药大学.
A105	陈演仪. (2010) 针刺配合康复疗法对中风病肢体痉挛患者的临床观察 (Thesis). 广州中医药大学.
A106	席朝垒. (2012) 针刺膀胱经穴位对中风偏瘫患者踝背屈功能的影响 (Thesis). 福建中医药大学.
A107	卢凤娟. (2011) 针刺经筋结点结合 Bobath 疗法治疗中风后痉挛性瘫痪的临床疗效观察 (Thesis). 黑龙江中医药大学.
A108	徐海艳. (2014) 针刺结合康复训练治疗中风恢复期足下垂的疗效观察 (Thesis). 黑龙江中医药大学.
A109	张雪艳. (2002) 针刺拮抗肌、艾灸痉挛肌配合康复训练治疗中风后肢体痉挛临床观察 (Thesis). 福建中医药大学.
A110	周穗萍. (2013) 穴位透刺结合康复疗法治疗脑卒中后足内翻患者的临床疗效 (Thesis). 广州中医药大学.

(*Continued*)

(*Continued*)

Study ID	References
A111	陈弘严. (2012) 全经针刺法结合康复训练治疗恢复期中风偏瘫痉挛状态的临床观察 (Thesis). 湖南中医药大学.
A112	孙海燕. (2003) 梅花针治疗中风偏瘫痉挛状态的研究 (Thesis). 北京中医药大学.
A113	张文立, 封丽华, 贾小红, 樊建平, 张子明. (2007) 透穴针刺治疗卒中后偏瘫痉挛状态的临床观察. 中国全科医学 **(12):** 1031–1032.
A114	张旭, 李奇辉, 李营营, 陈传帮, 卢君艳, 朱蓓蕾, 郑瑞献, 练纯, 叶天申. (2012) 针刺结合运动再学习早期干预对脑梗死患者肌张力及其运动功能的影响. 中华物理医学与康复杂志 **34(4):** 279–282.
A115	卢君艳. (2009) 对应与中轴针刺对偏瘫患者肌痉挛、运动功能及 ADL 的影响 (Thesis). 温州医学院.
A116	赵鑫. (2009) 头穴丛刺结合主被动智能运动训练器对脑梗死患者下肢功能的影响 (Thesis). 黑龙江中医药大学.
A117	周海云, 姬卫东, 王遂山, 张美英, 杨海峰, 温秀兰. (2009) 电针对脑卒中患者软瘫肢体肌张力及运动功能的影响. 中华物理医学与康复杂志 **31(6):** 400–403.
A118	金荣疆, 朱天民, 王倩. (2010) 电针拮抗肌腧穴复合易化技术对脑梗塞后偏瘫患者运动功能及日常生活能力的影响. 成都中医药大学学报 **33(3):** 9–12.
A119	王英姿, 何丽君, 王纯强. (2008) 电针拮抗肌穴位结合运动疗法治疗脑卒中后肌痉挛. 中外医疗 **27(23):** 17–18.
A120	姚国新, 曾科学, 周飞雄. (2012) 电针拮抗肌穴位结合运动疗法治疗脑卒中后肌痉挛. 按摩与康复医学 **3(9):** 19.
A121	褚瑰翔, 易小琴. (2009) 电针结合康复疗法治疗中风痉挛性瘫痪的临床观察. 湖北中医杂志 **31(8):** 13–14.
A122	于敏, 张辉. (2007) 电针结合康复训练改善偏瘫患者痉挛的疗效观察. 中国全科医学 **10(21):** 1803–1804.
A123	李红星, 岳国荣, 刘东坡, 周红芳. (2011) 电针结合康复训练治疗脑卒中后足下垂 30 例. 云南中医中药杂志 **32(6):** 70–71.
A124	于晋云, 郭兴富. (2009) 电针结合康复训练治疗脑卒中痉挛状态的疗效观察. 中医外治杂志 **18(4):** 42–43.
A125	吴北峰, 高维滨, 杨续艳, 李雪岩. (2008) 电针结合康复治疗脑卒中偏瘫肢体痉挛 30 例. 针灸临床杂志 **24(5):** 24–25.

(*Continued*)

(*Continued*)

Study ID	References
A126	樊留博, 马利中. (2011) 电针联合肌电生物反馈疗法对痉挛性偏瘫患者 h 波及 m 波的影响. 中华中医药杂志 **26(7):** 1624–1626.
A127	严伟, 霍文璟, 姚波, 殷建权. (2010) 电针联合运动疗法治疗脑梗死后肌痉挛的疗效观察. 中华物理医学与康复杂志 **32(2):** 139–141.
A128	公维军, 张通, 崔利华, 杨宇琦, 孙新亭. (2008) 电针足三里改善脑卒中偏瘫痉挛期患者下肢运动功能的临床研究. 中国康复理论与实践 **14(11):** 1057–1058.
A129	王仲明, 姚莹莹. (2014) 浮针缪刺法结合康复治疗中风后肢体痉挛疗效观察. 浙江中西医结合杂志 **24(10):** 888–890.
A130	王家颖, 欧阳八四. (2014) 恢刺结合康复训练对脑卒中后上肢偏瘫痉挛患者生活质量的影响. 成都中医药大学学报 **37(1):** 68–70.
A131	王家颖, 欧阳八四. (2013) 恢刺结合康复训练改善脑卒中后上肢偏瘫痉挛状态疗效观察. 山西中医 **29(11):** 37–38.
A132	冯晓东. (2007) 灸针并重治疗脑卒中后痉挛状态的疗效分析. 中医研究 **20(12):** 52–54.
A133	薛茜, 李淑萍, 霍国敏. (2008) 平衡肌张力针法对硬瘫期偏瘫患者运动功能康复的影响. 江苏中医药 **40(2):** 55–56.
A134	周璐, 谢辉, 陈锐, 何可, 刘小卫, 艾坤. (2013) 牵张训练配合 " 平衡阴阳 " 电针法治疗脑卒中痉挛期足内翻的临床观察. 湖南中医药大学学报 **33(11):** 90–92.
A135	陈勤, 陈晓军, 陈利芳, 王樟连. (2013) 调和阴阳针法治疗中风后痉挛性瘫痪30例疗效观察. 浙江中医杂志 **48(9):** 672–673.
A136	张慧敏, 唐强. (2011) 针刺加康复防治脑卒中异常运动模式的康复学评定. 中国针灸 **31(6):** 487–492.
A137	谷巍, 李翠艳, 金晓仙, 刘泰. (2013) 针刺治疗脑卒中后痉挛性偏瘫临床观察. 四川中医 **31(5):** 132–133.
A138	杨德福, 林兴栋, 于征淼, 吴智兵, 吴宣富, 林洁芬. (2007) 组合针刺结合 Bobath 疗法对脑卒中偏瘫痉挛状态及运动功能的影响. 辽宁中医杂志 **34(2):** 215–216.
A139	杨珩. (2007) 电针配合康复训练治疗脑梗死偏瘫肢体痉挛状态的临床观察 (Thesis). 黑龙江中医药大学.
A140	何坚. (2008) 不同频率电针治疗脑卒中下肢痉挛的表面肌电研究 (Thesis). 广州中医药大学.

(*Continued*)

(*Continued*)

Study ID	References
A141	李琳, 柳涛. (2010) 手指点穴对脑卒中偏瘫患者痉挛的早期干预. 吉林医学 **31(10):** 1400–1401.
A142	马玉强, 李斌, 徐士军, 李英华, 纪茹英. (2013) 运动疗法联用按压穴位对脑卒中上肢痉挛状态临床观察. 中国医刊 **48(9):** 89–90.
A143	潘智美, 谭凯文, 李洪波, 梁焕英. (2009) 自拟药棒循经推按法治疗中风后瘫肢痉挛的疗效观察. 广西中医药 **32(4):** 11–12.
A144	霍新慧, 赵百孝, 周钰, 黄海霞. (2013) 艾灸结合康复治疗对中风后痉挛性偏瘫患者生存质量的影响. 辽宁中医杂志 **40(12):** 2566–2567.
A145	徐玉梅, 刘燕平, 彭思萍, 陈玉清. (2013) 艾灸治疗中风后痉挛性偏瘫的疗效观察与护理. 中国实用医药 **8(14):** 195–196.
A146	李志燕, 易琼, 潘军, 丁敏. (2013) 大灸治疗中风后肢体痉挛状态的临床研究. 中医药导报 **19(6):** 55–57.
A147	冯晓东, 刘飞来, 郭青川, 宋晓蕾, 宋琳琳, 孙伟娟, 李瑞青. (2014) 益阳灸结合康复训练对脑卒中后肢体痉挛患者的疗效观察. 中国康复医学杂志 **29(11):** 1063–1065.
A148	霍新慧. (2014) 艾灸结合康复训练对脑卒中偏瘫痉挛状态的临床研究 (Thesis). 北京中医药大学.
A149	迟振海, 熊俊, 陈日新, 余航, 焦琳, 张衍辉, 杨海. (2013) 循经往返灸加反射抑制模式治疗脑卒中后痉挛性偏瘫患者 30 例临床研究. 中医杂志 **54(7):** 580–583.
A150	周莉, 施伟. (2014) 运动灸配合反射抑制模式治疗脑卒中后痉挛性瘫痪疗效评价. 上海针灸杂志 **33(6):** 533–535.
A151	姜京明, 岳增辉, 叶禹, 李良, 李向荣. (2010) 针刺缓解中风痉挛性瘫痪诊疗方案的临床研究. 中国中医药信息杂志 **17(10):** 14–16.
A152	薛茜, 熊国星, 霍国敏, 李淑萍. (2007) 电针阳明经穴位对偏瘫患者运动功能康复的影响. 中国康复理论与实践 **13(11):** 1056–1057.
A153	马云枝, 王维杰, 杨靖. (2010) 体针结合运动疗法治疗脑卒中后痉挛性瘫痪 36 例. 中医杂志 **51(12):** 1104–1105.
A154	程红亮, 李飞, 胡培佳, 张闻东, 陈幸生, 韩为. (2012) 通督调神针法治疗脑卒中后痉挛瘫期的临床研究. 中医药临床杂志 **24(6):** 499–501.
A155	唐强, 朱冬梅, 刘景隆, 张立国, 王艳, 徐波克. (2004) 头穴丛刺结合康复治疗急性脑梗死患者运动功能障碍的临床观察. 中国康复理论与实践 **10(11):** 697–698.

(*Continued*)

(***Continued***)

Study ID	References
A156	赵然, 张勇, 崔伟, 任秀云, 龚英峰. (2014) 盐酸乙哌立松联合去瘀生新针法治疗老年脑出血患者术后痉挛性瘫痪 42 例. 中国药业 **23(22):** 102–103.
A157	孙凡, 徐守宇, 解光尧, 石敏. (2014) 针刺夹脊穴结合康复训练对脑卒中患者下肢 H 反射的影响. 浙江中医杂志 **49(4):** 280–281.
A158	毛华, 金保山, 黄元奎, 高文宏, 陶亮. (2014) 针刺拮抗肌疗法与 Bobath 技术治疗脑出血后偏瘫痉挛状态 32 例临床观察. 中医药导报 **20(4):** 95–96.
A159	和婧伟. (2013) 针刺结合运动疗法治疗脑卒中致痉挛临床研究. 实用中医药杂志 **29(12):** 1040–1041.
A160	李东霞, 胡培佳, 程红亮, 李飞, 周婷. (2013) 针刺井穴治疗脑梗死后肢体痉挛临床研究. 中医药临床杂志 **25(11):** 999–1000.
A161	王正田. (2007) 针刺治疗脑卒中后上肢痉挛的疗效观察. 针灸临床杂志 **23(7):** 16–17.
A162	勾丽洁, 许士奇. (2007) 针灸辅助治疗脑卒中后肢体痉挛的疗效观察. 承德医学院学报 **24(2):** 156–157.
A163	郭文海, 王艳, 白震民. (2006) 针灸早期介入对脑梗塞后痉挛的影响. 中国伤残医学 **14(4):** 37.
A164	李勇, 吴思平. (2001) "甲角"穴治疗中风偏瘫上肢手指拘挛的疗效观察. 中国针灸 **21(4):** 211–212.
A165	蒋花, 王顺. 侯权峰. (2008) 苍龟探穴法针刺治疗中风后腕关节痉挛1例. 上海针灸杂志 **27(7):** 19.
A166	胡智慧, 顾晓园. (1999) 电针缓解中风偏瘫痉挛的疗效观察. 中国针灸 **(4):** 205–206.
A167	魏冰, 李岩. (2010) 电针治疗脑卒中后上肢痉挛性瘫痪 32 例. 针灸临床杂志 **26(6):** 40–41.
A168	郭泽新, 汪润生, 陈向华, 周美启, 王燕. (1995) 分部针刺治疗中风偏瘫痉挛 68 例临床观察. 中国针灸 **(5):** 7–8.
A169	何晓华. (2008) 恢刺和关刺法治疗中风后上肢痉挛性瘫痪临床观察. 上海中医药杂志 **42(12):** 45–46.
A170	高洁, 欧阳八四. (2007) 恢刺加电针对中风患者痉挛状态缓解的临床观察. 湖南中医杂志 **23(6):** 3–4.
A171	黄靖宇, 万娇, 钱俊辉, 罗才贵. (2009) 巨刺法治疗中风后上肢痉挛性瘫痪 45 例. 河南中医 **29(8):** 806–807.

(*Continued*)

(Continued)

Study ID	References
A172	黄靖宇, 万娇, 钱俊辉, 范宏元, 罗才贵. (2009) 巨刺法治疗中风后上肢痉挛性瘫痪 45 例疗效观察. 亚太传统医药 **5(1):** 74–75.
A173	王国书, 俞昌德. (2006) 颅体针结合治疗中风后痉挛瘫痪 35 例. 针灸临床杂志 **22(8):** 12–13.
A174	李政, 刘恩远. (2011) 平衡阴阳刺法治疗中风后上肢痉挛性瘫痪 50 例临床观察. 新疆中医药 **29(4):** 46–48.
A175	刘恩远, 马蕾, 李政. (2014) 平衡阴阳刺法治疗中风后上肢痉挛性瘫痪临床研究. 甘肃科技 **30(4):** 112–113, 171.
A176	金远林, 王海燕, 周启棣, 吴军君, 张莉梅. (2006) 祛瘀生新针法治疗中风后肢体痉挛 52 例临床观察. 光明中医 **21(3):** 40–41.
A177	柏玲, 范丽, 郑闵琴, 孙燕, 唐筱璐. (2008) 三间透后溪治疗中风后遗症手指痉挛. 中国针灸 2008 增刊 103.
A178	吴常征, 丁一, 焦杨. (2013) 头皮针加体针透刺治疗中风后痉挛性瘫痪 42 例. 光明中医 **28(11):** 2269, 2276.
A179	杨翊, 周光涛, 刘经星, 张德清. (2012) 头针配合电针治疗脑卒中痉挛性偏瘫 124 例. 上海针灸杂志 **31(3):** 171–172.
A180	吴芬芬, 武连仲, 孟智宏. (2012) 武连仲教授妙用"下极泉"治疗上肢痉挛性瘫痪. 针灸临床杂志 **28(11):** 63–65.
A181	冯春燕, 张春红, 武连仲. (2009) 武连仲教授运用极泉穴治疗上肢挛萎经验介绍. 新中医 **41(12):** 10.
A182	郭晓艳. (2013) 醒脑开窍法治疗中风后手挛萎 32 例疗效观察. 四川中医 **31(11):** 126–127.
A183	王明月. (2011) 醒脑开窍针刺法配合合谷穴透刺治疗脑卒中后手指痉挛. 长春中医药大学学报 **27(3):** 440–441.
A184	舒丽华, 蔡伟. (2012) 阳陵泉透刺阴陵泉治疗脑卒中后下肢痉挛状态的临床观察. 中医临床研究 **4(2):** 54–55.
A185	赵丹丹. (2010) 阴阳经合刺治疗中风后痉挛性偏瘫浅识. 实用中医内科杂志 **24(11):** 48–49.
A186	时国臣, 郑晓旭, 宋楠楠. (2015) 运动针刺经筋结点治疗中风后下肢痉挛性瘫 30 例. 中国针灸 **35(3):** 212.
A187	茅敏, 牟欣, 陈新. (2007) 针刺后溪穴治疗中风偏瘫上肢手指拘挛 40 例. 实用中医药杂志 **23(5):** 313.

(Continued)

(*Continued*)

Study ID	References
A188	龙佳佳, 庄小强, 言丽燕. (2012) 针刺肌筋膜触发点治疗中风后痉挛 50 例. 广西中医药大学学报 **15(4):** 38–39.
A189	陈敬君. (2002) 针刺手三阴经穴治疗脑卒中后偏瘫上肢拘挛的疗效观察. 中国临床康复 **6(1):** 118.
A190	王文礼, 张伟, 邹俊杰. (2014) 针刺腕骨穴对脑卒中后手指拘挛的影响. 中医外治杂志 **23(4):** 30–31.
A191	马臣, 崔旻, 李岚, 李芳华, 韩广云, 刘靖, 赵桂贤, 张会霞. (2008) 针刺治疗手指痉挛 60 例. 中国针灸 **28(11):** 804.
A192	姜诗谦, 王鹏. (2005) 针刺治疗中风后关节痉挛 60 例. 中华当代医学 **3(3):** 94–95.
A193	张艳. (2005) 针刺治疗中风后下肢痉挛状态临床观察. 针灸临床杂志 **21(5):** 9–10.
A194	陈华, 张昭, 闫晓瑞, 周建伟. (2008) 针刺治疗中风肢体痉挛症的临床观察. 辽宁中医杂志 **35(2):** 277–278.
A195	廖杏球. (2012) 针灸治疗脑卒中痉挛性偏瘫临床效果观察. 中外医疗 **31(11):** 141.
A196	杜琳, 张章, 韩义皇, 刘娜, 蔡承穆. (2013) 足印分析法评价针灸治疗中风痉挛步态疗效. 中国中医药信息杂志 **20(2):** 74–75.
A197	何晓华. (2005) 透刺法治疗中风后上肢痉挛状态的临床观察与机理探讨 (Thesis). 天津中医学院.
A198	赵晓峰. (2002) ‘补缓泻急’ 针刺法治疗中风后肢体肌痉挛的临床研究 (Thesis). 天津中医学院.

8

Clinical Evidence for Other Chinese Medicine Therapies

OVERVIEW

Along with Chinese herbal medicine and acupuncture therapies, other Chinese medicine therapies, such as traditional Chinese *tuina* 推拿, can be used clinically to treat post-stroke spasticity. Efficacy and safety data of 16 randomised controlled trials and one non-randomised controlled trial, as well as key information on three non-controlled clinical studies, were reviewed in this chapter; all of these studies evaluated traditional Chinese *tuina* 推拿 therapy. Overall, there is promising evidence available for traditional Chinese *tuina* 推拿 therapy for post-stroke spasticity.

Introduction

In addition to Chinese herbal medicine (CHM) and acupuncture therapies, Chinese medicine (CM) includes a range of other CM therapies including traditional Chinese *tuina* 推拿 therapy (Chinese remedial massage therapy) to treat disease and maintain health. This chapter evaluates the clinical evidence of other CM therapies for post-stroke spasticity. Data from randomised controlled trials (RCTs) and a non-randomised controlled trial were evaluated for efficacy and safety. Non-controlled clinical studies were summarised for key information of relevant treatments.

- Chinese remedial massage (*tuina* 推拿): Pressing and rubbing on meridians, acupuncture points, muscles and skin areas with different parts of the palms and fingers and varying degrees of force.

Previous Systematic Reviews

Our database search identified three meta-analysis publications[1–3]; all of them evaluated the efficacy of traditional Chinese *tuina* 推拿 therapy. Two articles were duplications of the same meta-analysis research.[2,3]

Yan *et al.* (2015) systematically reviewed 20 RCTs of traditional Chinese *tuina* 推拿 therapy for post-stroke spasticity which were published before April 2014.[1] A total of 1,720 participants were included in this review. All studies were conducted in China and published in the Chinese language. Risk of bias assessment was used for methodological quality evaluation. Overall quality of the included RCTs was 'low' to 'moderate'. The Modified Ashworth Scale (MAS), Fugl-Meyer Assessment (FMA) and Modified Bathel Index (MBI) were used as outcome measures to evaluate the treatment effects. Meta-analyses showed that *tuina* 推拿 therapy was superior to routine care for all three outcome measures: MAS (nine studies, standardised mean difference (SMD): −1.37 [−1.46, −1.28]), FMA (ten studies, mean difference (MD): 4.51 [2.74, 6.28]), and MBI (seven studies, MD: 10.08 [8.13, 12.04]). However, such meta-analyses did not separate studies of *tuina* 推拿 therapy compared to routine care from studies of *tuina* 推拿 therapy as an add-on to routine care for sub-group analysis.

Fan *et al.* (2016) evaluated 16 RCTs which were published before July 2014.[2,3] All studies were conducted in China and published in the Chinese language. A total of 1,098 participants were included in these RCTs. Risk of bias assessment and the Jadad scale were used for methodological quality evaluation. Except for three RCTs, all other studies were assessed as 'low' quality. The included 16 RCTs assessed the efficacy of *tuina* 推拿 therapy of four comparisons: *tuina* 推拿 therapy versus acupuncture, *tuina* 推拿 therapy versus routine rehabilitation, *tuina* 推拿 therapy as an add-on to acupuncture and *tuina* 推拿 therapy as on add-on to routine rehabilitation. The Ashworth Scale (AS), FMA, MBI, Neuropathy Disability Score (NDS) and Composite Spasticity Index (CSI) were used for treatment effects evaluation. Subgroup meta-analyses showed that the treatment effects of *tuina* 推拿 therapy was superior to that of control groups in terms of FMA (of seven subgroups), AS and the NDS scores (of four subgroups), MBI (of three subgroups) and CSI scores (of one subgroup). In terms of the main outcome measure for spasticity (AS), the review authors did not consider separating different scales in the meta-analysis. The authors pointed out that, although there seem to be some evidence of *tuina* 推拿 therapy, the 'low' quality of included studies prevented any conclusions being drawn.

Identification of Clinical Studies

In total, 16 RCTs (O1–O16), one non-randomised controlled trial (O17), and three non-controlled clinical studies (O18–O20) were included according to the inclusion criteria (Fig. 8.1). All 20 clinical studies investigated the effects of *tuina* 推拿 therapy. Of the 16 RCTs, four studies compared *tuina* 推拿 therapy with routine rehabilitation; 11 studies compared the combination of *tuina* 推拿 therapy with routine rehabilitation to routine rehabilitation alone; and one study was a three-armed study which compared both *tuina* 推拿 therapy and the combination to routine rehabilitation. One non-randomised controlled trial investigated the add-on effects of *tuina* 推拿 therapy to the combination of botulinum toxin (BTX) injection and rehabilitation. Three non-controlled clinical studies are also of *tuina* 推拿 therapy. In addition, three studies were identified using interventions not commonly practised outside of China; they will not be presented here.

Randomised Controlled Trials of *Tuina* 推拿 Therapy

Sixteen RCTs evaluated the efficacy and safety of *tuina* 推拿 therapy. One study (O1) was three-armed: *tuina* 推拿 therapy alone, routine care/rehabilitation alone and, combining *tuina* 推拿 and routine rehabilitation. Three RCTs (O2–O4) compared *tuina* 推拿 therapy to routine care/rehabilitation, and another 12 studies (O5–O16)

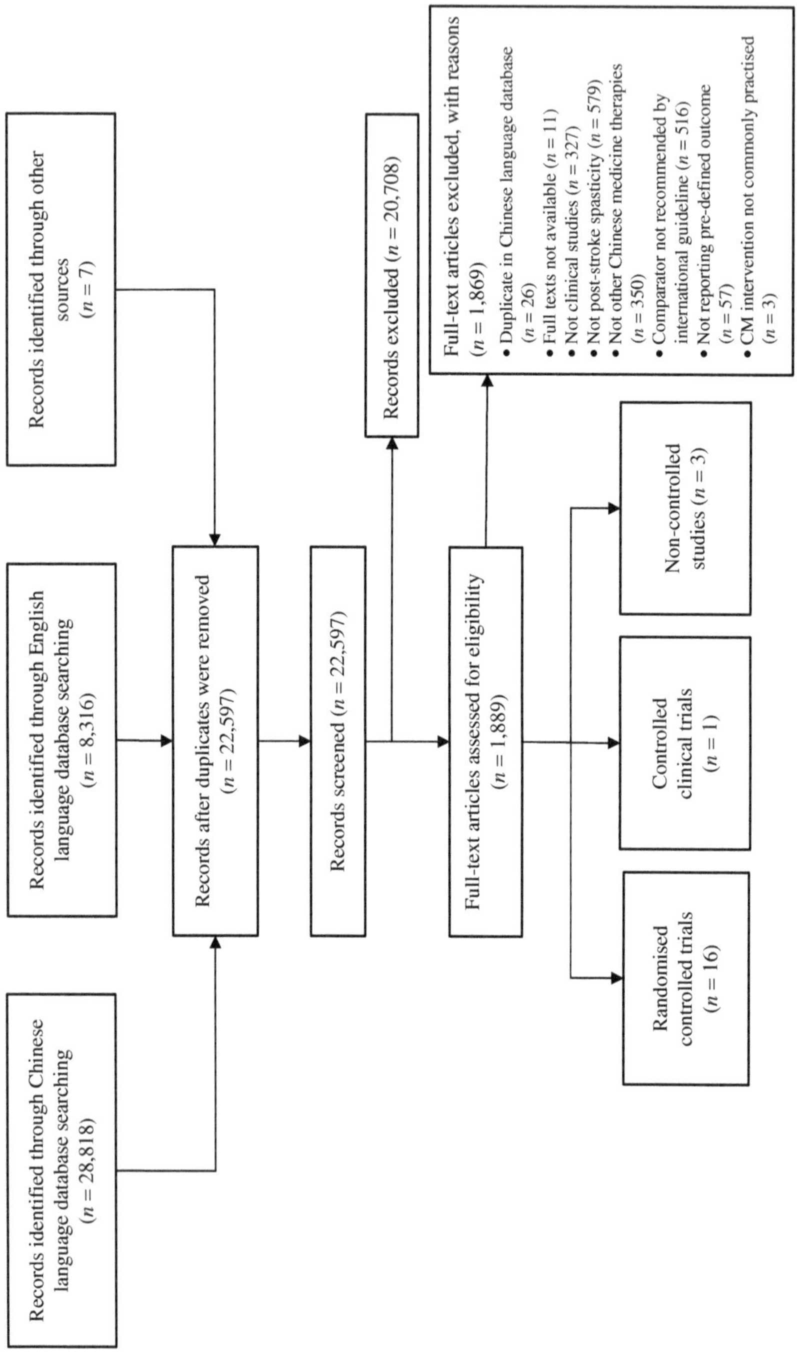

Fig. 8.1 Flowchart of study selection process: other Chinese medicine therapies.

compared the combination of *tuina* 推拿 therapy and routine care/rehabilitation to routine rehabilitation alone.

All RCTs were conducted in China, with participants recruited from the outpatient department alone, or from both inpatient and outpatient departments. A total of 1,139 participants were included in these studies. Of the studies that reported mean age, the average was 58.4 years. The studies included more males than females (331 and 273, respectively), although not all studies reported participants' gender, and some reported only for those who completed the study. The duration post-stroke ranged from five days (O1) to eight months (O6). None of the included RCTs reported using CM syndromes for either diagnosis or treatment. Detailed methods of *tuina* 推拿 therapy all varied, with muscles and acupuncture points of local areas being the focus. The common approach was to apply *tuina* 推拿 therapy one session each day, from ten to 50 minutes each time. The total treatment duration varied, with the longest one being three months (O8). The *tuina* 推拿 therapy methods involved multiple techniques as follows: pressing and rolling 按揉, kneading 提拿, applying finger pressure 点按, vigorous rubbing 搓摩 and rolling massage 㨰法. Eight RCTs (O5, O8, O10–O15) reported applying *tuina* 推拿 therapy techniques on various acupuncture points, with the most frequently used points being LI10 *Shousanli* 手三里 (n = 5), LI11 *Quchi* 曲池 (n = 5), LI15 *Jianyu* 肩髃 (n = 5), LI4 *Hegu* 合谷 (n = 4), ST5 *Waiguan* 外关 (n = 3), BL40 *Weizhong* 委中 (n = 3), HT3 *Shaohai* 少海 (n = 3) and GB30 *Huantiao* 环跳 (n = 3).

Risk of Bias Assessment of Included Randomised Controlled Trials

All included studies were described as 'randomised controlled trials'; four of them stated an appropriate method for randomisation sequence generation and therefore were assessed as 'low' risk of bias for this domain. One study used an incorrect method, thus it was 'high' risk of bias; the remaining studies were 'unclear' risk due to lack of information. For the allocation concealment, one RCT was 'low' risk of bias because it used the correct method; one study was

Table 8.1 Risk of Bias Assessment of Randomised Controlled Trials

Risk of Bias Domain	Low Risk *n* (%)	Unclear Risk *n* (%)	High Risk *n* (%)
Sequence generation	4 (25)	11 (68.8)	1 (6.3)
Allocation concealment	1 (6.3)	14 (87.5)	1 (6.3)
Blinding of participants	0 (0)	0 (0)	16 (100)
Blinding of personnel	0 (0)	0 (0)	16 (100)
Blinding of outcome assessors	0 (0)	16 (100)	0 (0)
Incomplete outcome data	16 (100)	0 (0)	0 (0)
Selective outcome reporting	0 (0)	16 (100)	0 (0)

Blinding of personnel (CM practitioner) is challenging in manual therapies.

'high' risk since the method was incorrect; the remaining studies were 'unclear' risk due to lack of information. Blinding of participants and personnel was judged as 'high' risk of bias in all studies because they were all designed to compare different treatments without any effort of blinding. Blinding of outcome assessors was all 'unclear' risk due to lack of information. Incomplete outcome data were assessed as 'low' risk of bias for all studies. All studies were assessed 'unclear' risk for selective reporting as protocols could not be identified for the studies. Overall the methodological quality was 'low', so results should be interpreted with caution. See Table 8.1 for a summary.

The treatment effects of *tuina* 推拿 therapy were evaluated according to pre-defined outcome measures.

Ashworth Scale or Modified Ashworth Scale

For the AS or MAS outcome, four studies (O10, O12, O15, O16) reported data of scores, and six studies (O2, O3, O5, O6, O9, O14) reported the number of people of each level. The results of the number of people were converted to corresponding scores for further analyses. On the occasion of studies reporting a different scoring system, SMD is used to present the results of meta-analyses.

Unspecified

One included study (O9) reported data on MAS (unspecified). Results showed that the combination of *tuina* 推拿 therapy and routine rehabilitation was superior to routine rehabilitation alone (MD: –0.53 [–0.70, –0.36]).

Upper Limb

MAS (upper limb) was reported by two RCTs (O2, O3) which compared *tuina* 推拿 therapy to routine rehabilitation alone; meta-analysis showed that *tuina* 推拿 therapy was more effective than routine rehabilitation (SMD: –0.56 [–0.84, –0.28], I^2 = 0%). Comparing the combination of *tuina* 推拿 therapy and routine rehabilitation to routine rehabilitation alone, three studies (O5, O6, O12) reported data on MAS (upper limb). Meta-analysis of these three studies showed that the combination was more effective than routine rehabilitation alone (SMD: –0.82 [–1.18, –0.46], I^2 = 0%).

Lower Limb

MAS (lower limb) was reported by one study (O2) which compared *tuina* 推拿 therapy to routine rehabilitation alone; the result showed that *tuina* 推拿 therapy was more effective than routine rehabilitation (MD: –0.41 [–0.73, –0.09]). Comparing the combination of *tuina* 推拿 therapy and routine rehabilitation to routine rehabilitation alone, three studies (O5, O14, O15) reported data on MAS (lower limb). Meta-analysis of these three studies showed that the combination was more effective than routine rehabilitation alone (SMD: –0.86 [–1.23, –0.50], I^2 = 0%).

Fugl-Meyer Assessment

In terms of the outcome of FMA, included studies reported data on FMA (motor), FMA (upper limb) or FMA (lower limb). Results were analysed for each outcome according to the comparison.

Motor

One three-armed study (O1) compared *tuina* 推拿 therapy, routine rehabilitation, and the combination of *tuina* 推拿 therapy and routine rehabilitation. When comparing *tuina* 推拿 therapy to routine rehabilitation (O1), the result showed that *tuina* 推拿 therapy was inferior to routine rehabilitation for FMA scores (motor function) (MD: –6.07 [–6.76, –5.38]). Furthermore, three studies (O1, O11, O15) comparing the combination of *tuina* 推拿 therapy and routine rehabilitation to routine rehabilitation alone also reported data on this outcome. It was found that the combination was more effective than routine rehabilitation alone (MD: 4.57 [3.05, 6.09], I^2 = 14%).

Upper Limb

Seven studies (O7, O8, O10, O12–O15) comparing the combination of *tuina* 推拿 therapy and routine rehabilitation, to routine rehabilitation alone, reported data on this outcome. Meta-analysis showed that the combination achieved greater effects than routine rehabilitation alone (MD: 4.85 [1.32, 8.38], I^2 = 83%); however, a high heterogeneity was detected. Once the study with 'high' risk of bias of randomisation (O8) was removed, the heterogeneity reduced to being 'moderate' with the treatment effects remaining in favour of the combination therapy (MD: 4.16 [0.45, 7.86], I^2 = 68%) (O7, O10, O12–O15).

Subgroup analysis was conducted based on the treatment duration. Seven studies were subgrouped as treatment: (1) less than 12 weeks (MD: 4.54 [0.83, 8.25], I^2 = 0%) (O7, O14, O15); and (2) 12 weeks or more (MD: 5.39 [0.58, 10.20], I^2 = 91%) (O8, O10, O12, O13). Both subgroups showed that the combination of *tuina* 推拿 therapy and routine rehabilitation was more effective than routine rehabilitation alone.

Lower Limb

Two studies (O14, O15) comparing the combination of *tuina* 推拿 therapy and routine rehabilitation, to routine rehabilitation alone, reported data on this outcome. Meta-analysis showed that there was no difference between the two groups (MD: 1.32 [–0.62, 3.25], $I^2 = 0\%$).

Barthel Index or Modified Barthel Index

Two studies (O1, O4) that compared *tuina* 推拿 therapy to routine rehabilitation reported data on MBI. Meta-analysis showed that there was no significant difference between these two therapies (MD: 0.20 [–16.21, 16.60], $I^2 = 97\%$), however, with a 'high' heterogeneity being detected. Taking the treatment duration into consideration, it was found that the study that applied longer treatment duration (four weeks) (O4) achieved greater effects in the *tuina* 推拿 therapy group (MD: 8.82 [3.10, 14.54]). In comparison, for the study that applied shorter treatment duration (ten days) (O1), the treatment effect was in favour of the routine rehabilitation (MD: –7.93 [–8.72, –7.14]).

Six studies (O1, O5–O7, O11, O14) comparing the combination of *tuina* 推拿 therapy and routine rehabilitation, to routine rehabilitation alone, also reported data on this outcome. Meta-analysis showed that adding *tuina* 推拿 therapy to routine rehabilitation was more effective than routine rehabilitation alone (MD: 10.22 [6.11, 14.32], $I^2 = 66\%$), with a moderate heterogeneity being detected. None of these studies were assessed as 'high' risk of bias of randomisation sequence generation; therefore the sensitivity analysis according to randomisation could not be performed. All six studies applied treatment for four weeks (or 30 days); hence subgroup analysis based on treatment duration is not feasible. All meta-analyses results are summarised in Table 8.2.

Assessment Using Grading of Recommendations Assessment, Development and Evaluation

Summary of findings tables were prepared for the comparisons of *tuina* 推拿 therapy plus rehabilitation versus rehabilitation alone. The evidence showed the benefit of adding *tuina* 推拿 therapy to rehabilitation for five outcomes: AS/MAS (upper limb), AS/MAS (lower

Table 8.2 Meta-analyses Results: *Tuina* 推拿 Therapy for Post-stroke Spasticity

Comparison	Outcomes	No. of studies	No. of participants	Effect size MD/ SMD [95% CI]	I² (%)	Included studies
Tuina 推拿 therapy versus routine rehabilitation	MAS (upper limb)	2	202	SMD: −0.56 [−0.84, −0.28]*	0	O2, O3
	MBI	2	165	MD: 0.20 [−16.21, 16.60]	97	O1, O4
Tuina 推拿 therapy plus routine rehabilitation versus routine rehabilitation alone	MAS (upper limb)	3	130	SMD: −0.82 [−1.18, −0.46]*	0	O5, O6, O12
	MAS (lower limb)	3	129	SMD: −0.86 [−1.23, −0.50]*	0	O5, O14, O15
	FMA (motor)	3	175	MD: 4.57 [3.05, 6.09]*	14	O1, O11, O15
	FMA (upper limb)	7	394	MD: 4.85 [1.32, 8.38]*	83	O7, O8, O10, O12–O15
	FMA (lower limb)	2	87	MD: 1.32 [−0.62, 3.25]	0	O14, O15
	MBI	6	332	MD: 10.22 [6.11, 14.32]*		O5–O7, O11, O14, O15

*Statistically significant.

Abbreviations: CI – confidence interval; FMA – Fugl-Meyer Assessment; MAS – Modified Ashworth Scale; MBI – Modified Barthel Index; MD – mean difference; SMD – standardised mean difference.

limb), FMA (motor function), FMA (upper limb) and BI were all assessed as 'low' certainty. See Table 8.3 for details.

Non-randomised Controlled Trials of *Tuina* 推拿 Therapy

One non-randomised controlled trial (O17) evaluated the add-on effects of *tuina* 推拿 therapy to BTX-injection plus routine rehabilitation. A total of 74 participants were included in this trial. Participants of more than six months after stroke onset, with an MAS level of 2–3 were included in this study. Thirty-six participants were assigned to receive the BTX-injection plus routine rehabilitation, and another 38 participants also received *tuina* 推拿 therapy in addition to the BTX-injection plus routine rehabilitation. *Tuina* 推拿 therapy was administered focusing on the muscles and acupuncture points located

Table 8.3 GRADE: *Tuina* 推拿 Therapy plus Rehabilitation Compared to Rehabilitation Alone for Post-stroke Spasticity

Outcomes	No. of Participants (Studies)	Certainty of the Evidence (GRADE)	Anticipated Absolute Effects	
			Risk with Rehabilitation	Risk Difference with *Tuina* 推拿 plus Rehabilitation
AS/MAS (upper limb)	130 (3 RCTs)	⊕⊕◯◯ LOW[a,b]	–	SMD **0.82 lower** (1.18 lower to 0.46 lower)
AS/MAS (lower limb)	129 (3 RCTs)	⊕⊕◯◯ LOW[a,b]	–	SMD **0.86 lower** (1.23 lower to 0.5 lower)
FMA (motor function)	175 (3 RCTs)	⊕⊕◯◯ LOW[a,b]	The mean FMA was **50.01** points.	MD **4.57 points higher** (3.05 higher to 6.09 higher)
FMA (upper limb)	394 (7 RCTs)	⊕⊕◯◯ LOW[a,c]	The mean FMA was **29.58** points.	MD **4.85 points higher** (1.32 higher to 8.38 higher)
FMA (lower limb)	87 (2 RCTs)	⊕⊕◯◯ LOW[a,b]	The mean FMA was **21.51** points.	MD **1.32 points higher** (0.62 lower to 3.25 higher)
MBI	332 (6 RCTs)	⊕⊕◯◯ LOW[a,b]	The mean MBI was **54.71** points.	MD **10.22 points higher** (6.11 higher to 14.32 higher)

The risk in the intervention group (and its 95% confidence interval) is based on the assumed risk in the comparison group and the **relative effect** of the intervention (and its 95% CI).

Abbreviations: AS – Ashworth Scale; BI – Barthel Index; CI – confidence interval; FMA – Fugl-Meyer Assessment; MAS – Modified Ashworth Scale; MD – mean difference; RCT – randomised controlled trial; SMD – standardised mean difference.

Notes
[a]Lack of blinding of participants, personnel and assessors.
[b]Small sample size limits certainty of results.
[c]Considerable statistical heterogeneity.

Study References
AS/MAS (upper limb): O5, O6, O12
AS/MAS (lower limb): O5, O14, O15
FMA (motor): O1, O11, O15
FMA (upper limb): O7, O8, O10, O12–O15
FMA (lower limb): O14, O15
BI: O5–O7, O11, O14, O15

on the diseased upper limb, for 20 to 30 minutes each session, five sessions each week. The total duration of treatment for both groups was 12 weeks.

Treatment effects were evaluated using MAS, FMA (upper limb) and MBI. The results show that adding *tuina* 推拿 therapy is more effective than the BTX-injection plus routine rehabilitation for FMA (upper limb) (MD: 3.29 [2.63, 3.95]). However, there was no significant difference for the other two outcomes: MAS (MD: –0.06 [–0.23, 0.11]) and MBI (MD: 4.70 [–4.36, 13.76]). Adverse events information was not mentioned by this study.

Non-controlled Clinical Studies of *Tuina* 推拿 Therapy

Three non-controlled clinical studies (O18–O20) were identified through the search; one study was a single case report (O18) and the other two were case series (O19, O20). All studies assessed *tuina* 推拿 therapy for post-stroke spasticity. A total of 77 participants were included in the three studies.

One case series study (O19) recruited patients with upper limb post-stroke spasticity and reported that *tuina* 推拿 therapy was conducted on acupuncture points located on the shoulder and arms. One case report (O18) reported details of the *tuina* 推拿 therapy applied to patient's upper limb with a focus on acupuncture points: HT1 *Jiquan* 极泉, LU5 *Chize* 尺泽, LI11 *Quchi* 曲池, LI10 *Shousanli* 手三里, LU6 *Kongzui* 孔最 and PC6 *Neiguan* 内关. The other study (O20) did not detail the information of *tuina* 推拿 therapy. All three studies concluded that *tuina* 推拿 therapy was effective for post-stroke spasticity; however, the effects were not compared to any control method. No adverse events were reported by any of the three studies.

Safety of *Tuina* 推拿 Therapy

None of the included studies reported information on adverse events. The safety of *tuina* 推拿 therapy for post-stroke spasticity is unclear. Further clinical research should take this aspect into consideration.

Evidence for Other Chinese Medicine Therapies Commonly Used in Clinical Practice

Tuina 推拿 therapy has been recommended by a clinical guideline for the treatment of post-stroke shoulder complications (see Chapter 2). It is suggested that *tuina* 推拿 therapy could emphasise antagonistic muscle groups to improve the recovery of myodynamia.

Our review found that the effects of *tuina* 推拿 therapy for post-stroke spasticity has been synthesised by a few systematic reviews, and also been evaluated by a number of clinical studies. Two meta-analysis studies suggested that *tuina* 推拿 therapy was effective for post-stroke spasticity; however, both studies suffered methodological weaknesses in their analysis. Sixteen RCTs were included in our evaluation. There is promising evidence from RCTs supporting the use of *tuina* 推拿 therapy for improving spasticity, in terms of the main outcome measure of MAS, when it was used as an add-on therapy to routine rehabilitation. Assessing motor function using FMA, our meta-analysis showed that adding *tuina* 推拿 therapy to routine rehabilitation is beneficial in improving upper limb motor function; however, this is not the case for the lower limb. Nevertheless, such a conclusion could not be drawn since there were only two studies included in the meta-analysis for FMA (lower limb). For patients' daily activity, our meta-analysis of six studies also supports that adding *tuina* 推拿 therapy to routine rehabilitation could significantly improve patients' daily activity (assessed by MBI).

Among all included studies, *tuina* 推拿 therapy was usually applied along meridians, with or without focusing on acupuncture points. Most of the included studies stated that attention should be paid to the strength of applying *tuina* 推拿 therapy on different muscles. A number of studies (O5, O7–O16) suggested that strong stimulation on the spasm muscles should be avoided.

Summary of Other Chinese Medicine Therapies Clinical Evidence

Our review of clinical studies found that *tuina* 推拿 therapy, when used as an add-on therapy to routine rehabilitation, is beneficial for reducing spasticity of upper limb (MAS upper limb) and lower limb (MAS lower limb). In addition, it improves patients' overall motor function (FMA motor) or upper limb motor function (FMA upper limb), as well as patients' daily activity (MBI). These findings are consistent with previously published systematic reviews.[1–3] However, evidence of the benefit of adding *tuina* 推拿 therapy to rehabilitation for five outcomes — AS or MAS (upper limb), AS or MAS (lower limb), FMA (motor function), FMA (upper limb) or MBI — were all assessed as 'low' certainty.

Tuina 推拿 therapy could be conducted daily for 10 to 50 minutes each time. Chinese medicine syndrome differentiation does not seem essential when applying *tuina* 推拿 therapy for the treatment of post-stroke spasticity since none of the included studies highlighted such information. *Tuina* 推拿 therapy could be applied on affected muscles, along meridians or focusing on certain acupuncture points. It is worth noting that the benefit of adding *tuina* 推拿 therapy to routine rehabilitation was seen in the study that applied treatment for four weeks; however, it was not seen in the study that used only ten days of this approach. This may indicate that longer treatment duration is needed when considering *tuina* 推拿 therapy in clinical practice. Nevertheless, more evidence is needed to confirm such a hypothesis.

References

1. 严连凤, 励建安, 朱毅, 马鑫, 金宏柱. (2015) 推拿治疗脑卒中后痉挛的 Meta 分析. 中国中医基础医学杂志 **21(12):** 1566–1568.
2. 范江华, 黄永, 王开龙, 马甜, 雷龙鸣. (2016) 从循证医学角度分析推拿治疗中风后痉挛性偏瘫的疗效. 中国中医基础医学杂志 **22(2):** 242–248.
3. 王开龙, 黄永, 范江华. (2016) 推拿治疗脑卒中痉挛状态的 meta 分析. 中国民族民间医药 **25(3):** 24–29.

References to Included Clinical Studies

Study ID	References
O1	郑智元. (2012) 疏经通督手法结合 Bobath 疗法对脑卒中康复效应的研究 (Thesis). 南京中医药大学.

(*Continued*)

(***Continued***)

Study ID	References
O2	陈群. (2010) 康复运动疗法治疗脑卒中后偏瘫肌痉挛的效果观察. 护理研究 **24(1):** 14–16.
O3	郑鹏, 徐晓红, 张为民, 王健. (2013) 推拿手法治疗中风后肘关节屈曲痉挛的临床观察. 世界科学技术,中医药现代化 **15(5):** 1029–1031.
O4	汤俊玲, 韩淑凯. (2011) 循经推拿治疗脑卒中后上肢痉挛疗效观察. 护理研究 **25(20):** 1839–1840.
O5	迟相林, 郭兆荣, 王道珍, 李振光, 詹霞. (2008) 联合中医按摩及神经促通技术治疗脑卒中后偏瘫肢体痉挛的疗效观察. 中华物理医学与康复杂志 **30(04):** 282–284.
O6	余天智, 李昌柳, 吕泽平, 庞国防, 李洁. (2011) 躯干扳法治疗痉挛性偏瘫的效果观察. 广西医学 **(7):** 821–823.
O7	杨冬梅. (2009) 手臂三阴经推拿治疗中风后上肢痉挛的疗效观察及护理. 护士进修杂志 **24(22):** 2052–2053.
O8	雷迈, 吕泽平, 谭威. (2012) 推拿点穴联合康复治疗对脑卒中偏瘫患者上肢功能恢复的影响. 广西医学 **34(12):** 1613–1615.
O9	何炯. (2009) 推拿结合康复训练治疗脑卒中后痉挛疗效观察. 中国中医急症 **18(1):** 27–28.
O10	詹蕾, 张玉娟. (2012) 推拿与抗痉挛技术改善卒中患者肌痉挛的疗效. 上海护理 **12(5):** 21–23.
O11	林红霞, 廖辉雄, 王文靖. (2013) 现代康复训练结合中医按摩治疗脑卒中偏瘫痉挛状态疗效观察. 吉林中医药 **(4):** 99–101.
O12	陈峰, 苏庆军. (2011) 穴位推拿结合抗痉挛技术对脑卒中后上肢肌痉挛改善的疗效观察. 中国实用神经疾病杂志 **14(1):** 74–75.
O13	詹蕾, 吴璇, 廖阳. (2012) 穴位推拿结合抗痉挛技术抑制脑卒中患者上肢肌痉挛疗效观察. 新乡医学院学报 **29(3):** 201–203.
O14	王亚锋. (2003) 中医按摩结合现代康复训练对中风病偏瘫痉挛状态的疗效观察. (Thesis). 北京中医药大学.
O15	王海宽. (2014) 推拿结合 Bobath 疗法治疗中风后痉挛性瘫痪的疗效观察. (Thesis). 广州中医药大学.
O16	彭进. (2013) 两步十法推拿结合康复训练治疗中风偏瘫痉挛状态患者的疗效观察. (Thesis). 北京中医药大学.
O17	秦茵, 崔利华, 郭健红. (2012) 中医推拿对脑卒中后上肢痉挛 a 型肉毒毒素干预效果的影响. 中国康复理论与实践 **18(12):** 1109–1111.
O18	左贾逸. (2015) 放松训练手法在推拿治疗脑卒中痉挛性瘫痪中的应用体会. 科技展望 **(01):** 239.

(*Continued*)

(*Continued*)

Study ID	References
O19	魏乾坤, 闫玮娟, 楚燕萍, 李桂粉, 代新年. (2012) 手法与徒手牵引相结合治疗脑卒中后上肢痉挛临床观察. 中国疗养医学 **(7):** 627–628.
O20	刘海潮, 蒋惠瑜. (2009) 推拿结合运动疗法缓解偏瘫痉挛 40 例观察. 中国康复理论与实践 **15(6):** 588.

9

Clinical Evidence for Chinese Medicine Combined Therapies

OVERVIEW

Clinical practice of Chinese medicine often sees several therapy types used in combination, such as Chinese herbal medicine plus acupuncture. Twenty-eight randomised controlled trials, which used combinations of Chinese medicine therapies, were reviewed in this chapter. The most common combination was Chinese herbal medicine with acupuncture therapies. The results showed benefits for the majority of combinations.

Introduction

The practice of using two or more different Chinese medicine (CM) interventions together is common in the clinical management of post-stroke spasticity. Such combinations included Chinese herbal medicine (CHM) with acupuncture, CHM with *tuina* 推拿 therapy, or acupuncture and *tuina* 推拿 therapy. In this chapter, combinations of CM therapies were identified from literature searches, and randomised controlled trials (RCTs) were examined to evaluate their efficacy and safety.

Identification of Clinical Studies

In total 28 RCTs (C1 to C28), including 2,705 participants, were selected according to the inclusion criteria (Fig. 9.1). Of these, three

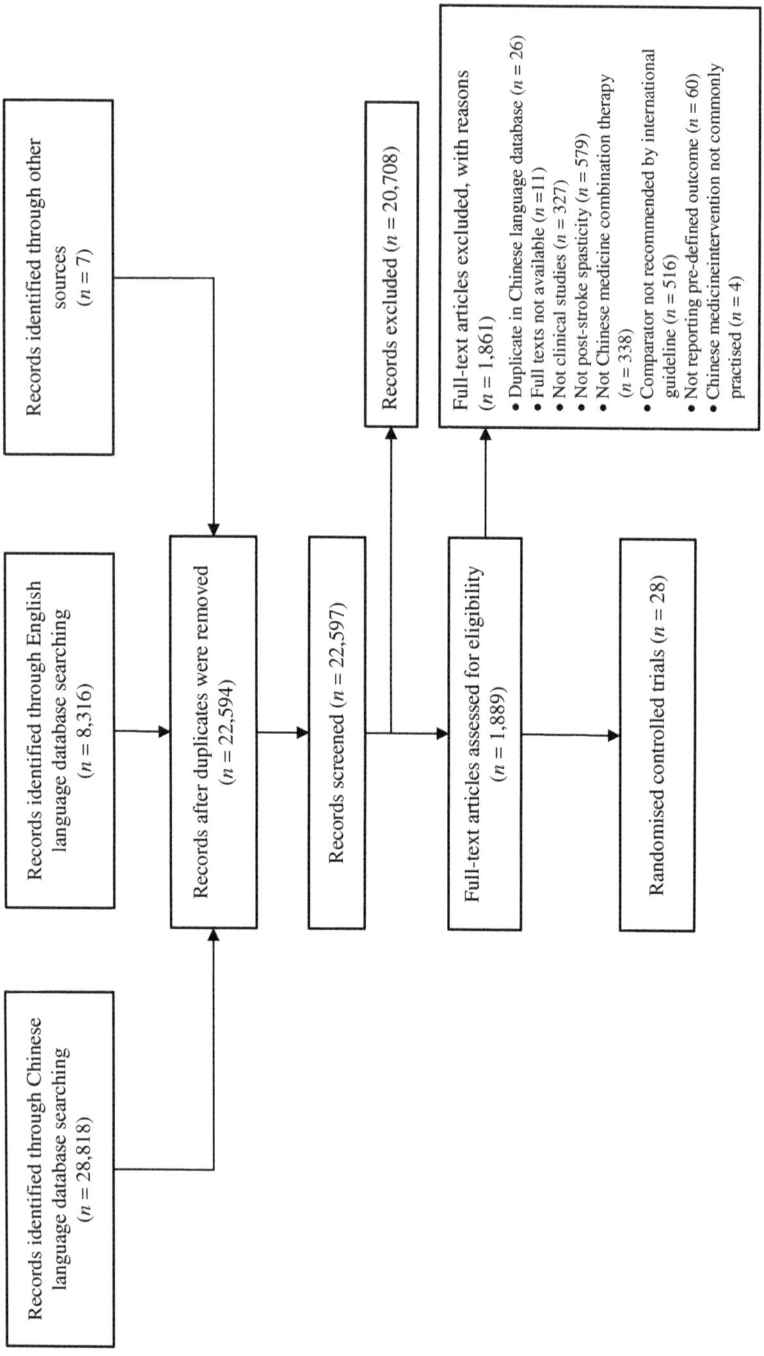

Fig. 9.1 Flowchart of study selection process: Chinese medicine combination therapies.

studies (C1–C3) compared CM combination therapies to routine care/rehabilitation and 25 RCTs (C4–C28) compared CM combination therapies plus routine care/rehabilitation to routine care/rehabilitation alone. Studies were conducted in China, in outpatient departments or both inpatient and outpatient departments. The studies included more males than females (1,112 and 783, respectively), although not all studies reported participant's gender, and some reported only for those who completed the study.

The age of participants ranged from 46 to 76 years, and in studies which reported the mean age, the median of the mean age was 48.9 years. The duration of post-stroke spasticity ranged from 14 days (C3) to 12 months (C12). Follow-up assessment after the treatment phase was only conducted in two studies (C11, C27). Four studies (C11, C13, C16, C27) reported using CM syndromes for either diagnosis, treatment, or both. All these four studies reported multiple syndromes, the common syndromes including *qi* deficiency, Blood stasis and Phlegm stagnation.

Therapies used in these studies were CHM, acupuncture, moxibustion, cupping therapy and *tuina* 推拿 therapy. Studies were grouped as seven combinations, the most common one being CHM plus acupuncture, which was tested in 20 RCTs. See Table 9.1 for a summary.

Table 9.1 Summary of Interventions in Combination Therapy Studies

Combination Therapies	No. of Studies	Included Studies
CHM plus acupuncture	20	C1–C5, C6, C7, C10–C15, C17–C19, C22, C24, C26, C27
CHM plus acupuncture plus *tuina* 推拿 therapy	4	C9, C21, C23, C25
CHM plus acupuncture plus moxibustion plus *tuina* 推拿 therapy	1	C16
CHM plus acupressure plus cupping therapy	1	C28
CHM plus *tuina* 推拿 therapy	2	C8, C20

Abbreviation: CHM – Chinese herbal medicine.

The most commonly used therapy was CHM, which was applied by all included studies (C1–C28). Among them, three studies used more than two CHM formulas (C11, C25, C28). Two formulas or products had been used in multiple studies; they were *Bu yang huan wu tang* 补阳还五汤, used in three studies (C2, C6, C13), and *Zhong feng hui chun wan* 中风回春丸, used by two studies (C14, C17). A total of 56 herbs were used in all formulas. The most frequently reported herbs were *chuan xiong* 川芎, *bai shao/chi shao* 白芍/赤芍, *dan shen* 丹参, *shui zhi* 水蛭, *huang qi* 黄芪, *hong hua* 红花 and *gan cao* 甘草 (Table 9.2).

Twenty-five studies (C1–C7, C9–C19, C21–C27) utilised acupuncture as a treatment. Of these, four studies (C5, C6, C19, C24) also applied scalp acupuncture in combination with body acupuncture. The most common acupuncture points used in these studies were LI4 *Hegu* 合谷, LI11 *Quchi* 曲池, ST36 *Zusanli* 足三里, SP6 *Sanyinjiao* 三阴交, LI10 *Shousanli* 手三里, LI15 *Jianyu* 肩髃, GB34 *Yanglingquan* 阳陵泉 and SP9 *Yinlingquan* 阴陵泉 (Table 9.3).

In addition, seven RCTs were identified for interventions not commonly practised outside of China; they are not presented here.

Risk of Bias Assessment

All included studies were described as RCTs; four of them stated an appropriate method for randomisation sequence generation and therefore were assessed as 'low' risk of bias for this domain. One study used an incorrect method, thus it was 'high' risk of bias and the remaining studies were 'unclear' risk due to lack of information. For the allocation concealment, one RCT was 'low' risk of bias because it used the correct method. One study was 'high' risk since the method was incorrect and the remaining studies were 'unclear' risk due to lack of information. Blinding of participants and personnel was judged as 'high' risk of bias in all studies because they were all designed to compare different treatments without any effort of blinding. Blinding of outcome assessors was all 'unclear' risk due to lack

Table 9.2 Frequently Reported Herbs in Combination Therapies Clinical Studies

Most Common Herbs	Scientific Name	Frequency of Use
Chuan xiong 川芎	*Ligusticum chuangxiong* Hort.	10
Bai shao/chi shao 白芍/赤芍	*Paeonia lactiflora* Pall.	10
Dan shen 丹参	*Salvia miltiorrhiza* Bge.	8
Shui zhi 水蛭	1. *Whitmania pigra* Whitman 2. *Hirudo nipponica* Whitman 3. *Whitmania acranulata* Whitman	7
Huang qi 黄芪	*Astragalus membranaceus* (Fisch.) Bge. var. *mongholicus* (Bge.) Hsiao / *Astragalus membranaceus* (Fisch.) Bge.	7
Hong hua 红花	*Carthamus tinctorius* L.	7
Gan cao 甘草	*Glycyrrhiza uralensis* Fisch./*Glycyrrhiza inflata* Bat./*Glycyrrhiza glabra* L.	7
Di long 地龙	*Pheretima aspergillum* (E. Perrier) / *Pheretima vulgaris* Chen/*Pheretima guillelmi* (Michaelsen)	6
Dang gui 当归	Angelica sinensis (Oliv.) Diels	5
Tao ren 桃仁	*Prunus persica* (L.) Batsch/*Prunus davidiana* (Carr.) Franch.	5
Hai feng teng 海风藤	*Chaenomeles speciosa* (Sweet) Nakai	5
Mu gua 木瓜	*Chaenomeles speciosa* (Sweet) Nakai	4
Sheng di huang 生地黄	*Rehmannia glutinosa* Libosch.	3
Shen jin cao 伸筋草	*Lycopodium japonicum* Thunb.	3
Ji xue teng 鸡血藤	*Spatholobus suberectus* Dunn	3
Mang chong 虻虫	1. *Tabanus mandarinus Schiner* 2. *Atylotus bivittateinus Takahasi*	3
Fu ling 茯苓	*Poria cocos (Schw.)* Wolf	2
San qi 三七	*Panax notoginseng* (Burk.) F. H. Chen	2
Jiang can 僵蚕	1. *Bombyx mori* L. 2. *Beauveria bassiana* (Bals.)	2
Quan xie 全蝎	*Buthus martensii* Karsch	2
Da zao 大枣	*Ziziphus jujuba* Mill.	2
Tian ma 天麻	*Gastrodia elata* Bl.	2
Shi chang pu 石菖蒲	*Acorus tatarinowii* Schott	2

Table 9.3 Frequently Used Points/Treatment Approaches in Combination Therapies from Clinical Studies

Most Common Points	No. of Studies
LI4 *Hegu* 合谷	16
LI11 *Quchi* 曲池	13
ST36 *Zusanli* 足三里	13
SP6 *Sanyinjiao* 三阴交	10
LI10 *Shousanli* 手三里	8
LI15 *Jianyu* 肩髃	8
GB34 *Yanglingquan* 阳陵泉	8
SP9 *Yinlingquan* 阴陵泉	8
PC6 *Neiguan* 内关	7
ST41 *Jiexi* 解溪	7
TE14 *Jianliao* 肩髎	6
SP10 *Xuehai* 血海	6
KI6 *Zhaohai* 照海	6
KI3 *Taixi* 太溪	6
BL40 *Weizhong* 委中	6
GB39 *Xuanzhong* 悬钟	6
GB40 *Qiuxu* 丘墟	5
BL57 *Chengshan* 承山	5
GB31 *Fengshi* 风市	5

of information. Incomplete outcome data were assessed as 'low' risk of bias for 27 studies, except for one study which did not report data on drop-out cases and thus it was assessed as 'high' risk. Two studies were assessed as 'high' risk of bias for selective reporting because it did not report data on the outcomes stated in its methodology section. The others were 'unclear' risk as protocols could not be identified for the studies. Overall the methodological quality was 'low' and therefore the results should be interpreted with caution. See Table 9.4 for a summary.

Table 9.4 Risk of Bias Assessment of Randomised Controlled Trials

Risk of Bias Domain	Low Risk *n* (%)	Unclear Risk *n* (%)	High Risk *n* (%)
Sequence generation	4 (14.3)	23 (82.1)	1 (3.6)
Allocation concealment	1 (3.6)	26 (90)	1 (3.6)
Blinding of participants	0 (0)	0 (0)	28 (100)
Blinding of personnel	0 (0)	0 (0)	28 (100)
Blinding of outcome assessor	0 (0)	28 (100)	0 (0%)
Incomplete outcome assessment	27 (96.4)	0 (0)	1 (3.6)
Selective reporting	0 (0)	26 (92.8)	2 (7.1)

Oral Chinese Herbal Medicine plus Acupuncture

Modified Ashworth Scale

Unspecified

Three studies (C5, C11, C17) evaluated the combination of oral CHM, acupuncture and rehabilitation compared to rehabilitation alone. Meta-analysis showed that adding oral CHM and acupuncture was not superior to rehabilitation alone for the outcome of Modified Ashworth Scale (MAS) (standardised mean difference (SMD): –1.08 [–2.30, 0.15], I^2 = 94%).

Upper Limb

Results from one study (C1) that compared oral CHM to routine rehabilitation showed that oral CHM was superior to rehabilitation at the end of treatment for upper limb MAS score (mean difference (MD): –0.93 [–1.33, –0.53]). Two studies (C6, C12) evaluated the combination of topical CHM, acupuncture and rehabilitation compared to rehabilitation alone. Both studies showed the benefit of the integrated therapy. It was found, by meta-analysis, that the integrated therapy was superior to rehabilitation alone (SMD: –0.92 [–1.29, –0.55], I^2 = 0%).

Fugl-Meyer Assessment

Motor

One study (C2) compared oral CHM plus acupuncture to medication (baclofen) alone. Results reported by this study showed that oral CHM combined with acupuncture was more effective than baclofen (MD: 10.33 [6.22, 14.44]).

Seven studies (C4, C12–C14, C19, C24, C27) used CHM plus acupuncture as an add-on therapy. Overall meta-analysis showed benefit of adding CHM plus acupuncture (MD: 19.66 [15.87, 23.44], I^2 = 50%). Subgroup analyses was conducted according to different treatments and showed that there was no benefit of adding oral CHM plus acupuncture to pharmacotherapy alone (MD: 15.68 [–2.40, 33.77], I^2 = 72%) (C4, C19). Adding oral CHM plus acupuncture to rehabilitation was more effective than rehabilitation alone (MD: 19.79 [14.93, 24.65], I^2 = 53%) (C13, C14, C24, C27). One study (C12) used topical CHM plus acupuncture; it was found that the integrative therapy was more effective than rehabilitation alone (MD: 21.79 [17.43, 26.15]).

Upper Limb

Six studies (C5, C11, C17, C18, C22, C26) evaluating the add-on effects of CHM plus acupuncture to rehabilitation reported data on Fugl-Myer Assessment (FMA — upper limb). It is noted that one study (C5) reported wrong data on this outcome and therefore it was not pooled in the meta-analysis. Two studies reported simplified versions of FMA with the total score of FMA (upper limb) being 36 points; therefore we used SMD to present the meta-analysis results. Overall meta-analysis of five studies (C11, C17, C18, C22, C26) showed benefit of adding CHM and acupuncture to rehabilitation (SMD: 1.18 [0.45, 1.90], I^2 = 90%).

Subgroup analyses found that when CHM was used both orally and topically, the integrative therapy was more effective than rehabilitation (SMD: 0.89 [0.05, 1.72], I^2 = 90%) (C18, C22, C26); a similar result was also found from the studies that used CHM only orally (MD: 11.03 [6.04, 16.01], I^2 = 62%) (C11, C17).

Lower Limb

Six studies (C5, C11, C17, C18, C22, C26) evaluating the add-on effects of CHM plus acupuncture to rehabilitation reported data on FMA (lower limb); one of these studies (C5) reported wrong data for this outcome and therefore it was not pooled in meta-analyses. Two studies (C22, C26) used a simplified version of FMA (lower limb) which uses 18 as the total score, therefore we used SMD to present the results of the meta-analysis. Overall meta-analysis of five studies (C11, C17, C18, C22, C26) showed benefit of adding CHM and acupuncture to rehabilitation (SMD 0.53 [0.33, 0.74], I^2 = 0%).

Subgroup analysis found that when CHM was used both orally and topically, the integrative therapy was more effective than rehabilitation (SMD: 0.51 [0.26, 0.75], I^2 = 0%) (C18, C22, C26). However, such results were not found from the studies that used CHM only orally (MD: 2.67 [–1.69, 7.03], I^2 = 85%) (C11, 17).

Barthel Index

One study (C1) compared oral CHM plus acupuncture to routine rehabilitation; there was no difference between these two treatments (MD: 11.46 [–11.88, 34.80]). Results from another single study (C2) showed that oral CHM plus acupuncture was superior to medication (baclofen) (MD: 12.97 [7.51, 18.43]).

Ten studies (C4–C6, C10, C11, C13, C17–C19, C27) used CHM plus acupuncture as add-on therapy. Three studies (C4, C10, C19) added oral CHM and acupuncture to pharmacotherapy. It was found that the integrated therapy was more effective than pharmacotherapy alone (MD: 20.32 [11.60, 29.05], I^2 = 79%). Seven studies (C5, C6, C11, C13, C17, C18, C27) compared the combination of CHM, acupuncture and rehabilitation to rehabilitation alone. It was found that the integrated therapy was more effective than rehabilitation alone

(MD: 12.87 [9.37, 16.37], I^2 = 55%). Subgroup analysis showed that adding oral CHM and acupuncture to rehabilitation was beneficial (MD: 10.78 [7.23, 14.33], I^2 = 28%) (C5, C11, C13, C17, C27). Furthermore, two single studies also showed benefit of adding topical CHM and acupuncture (MD: 14.00 [9.41, 18.59]) (C6), and adding both oral and topical CHM plus acupuncture (MD: 19.20 [13.20, 25.20]) (C18).

Safety of Oral Chinese Herbal Medicine plus Acupuncture

Four of 20 studies (C3, C11, C13, C27) reported information of adverse events. Three of them (C11, C13, C27) reported that there were no adverse events in both groups. One study (C3) reported adverse events from both groups; they are nausea (1 case) and muscle pain (three cases) reported from the oral CHM plus acupuncture group; nausea and dry mouth (two cases), dizziness and fatigue (five cases), and diarrhoea or constipation (three cases) reported from the pharmacotherapy (baclofen) group.

Chinese Herbal Medicine plus Acupuncture plus *Tuina* 推拿 Therapy

Four studies (C9, C21, C23, C25) evaluated the add-on effects of CHM, acupuncture and *tuina* 推拿 therapy to rehabilitation alone. Of them, two studies (C9, C21) used topical CHM and the other two (C23, C25) used both oral and topical CHM. Meta-analysis was not feasible because the studies did not report data on common outcome measures. It was found that the integrated therapy was more effective than rehabilitation alone for MAS (non-specified) (MD: –0.73 [–1.11, –0.35]) (C25), MAS (upper limb) (MD: –0.26 [–0.49, –0.03]) (C23) and Modified Barthel Index (MBI) (MD: 14.79 [11.99, 17.59]) (C21). However, such results were not seen in MAS (lower limb) (MD: –0.17 [–0.40, 0.06]) (C23). Adverse events data were not reported by these studies.

Table 9.5 Meta-analyses Results: Chinese Herbal Medicine plus Acupuncture

Comparison	Outcome Measure	No. of Studies	No. of Participants	Effect Size [95% CI]	I^2 (%)	Included Studies
Oral CHM plus acupuncture plus rehabilitation versus rehabilitation	AS or MAS (non-specified)	3	244	SMD: −1.08 [−2.30, 0.15]	94	C5, C11, C17
	FMA (motor)	4	330	MD: 19.79 [14.93, 24.65]*	53	C13, C14, C24, C27
	FMA (upper limb)	2	120	MD: 11.03 [6.04, 16.01]*	62	C11, C17
	FMA (lower limb)	2	120	MD: 2.67 [−1.69, 7.03]	85	C11, C17
	BI	5	354	MD: 10.78 [7.23, 14.33]*	28	C5, C11, C13, C17, C27
Oral CHM plus acupuncture plus pharmacotherapy versus pharmacotherapy	FMA (motor)	2	176	MD: 15.68 [−2.40, 33.77]	72	C4, C19
	BI	3	276	MD: 20.32 [11.60, 29.05]*	79	C4, C10, C19
Topical CHM plus acupuncture plus rehabilitation versus rehabilitation	AS or MAS (upper limb)	2	127	SMD: −0.92 [−1.29, −0.55]*	0	C6, C12
Oral CHM and topical CHM plus acupuncture plus rehabilitation versus rehabilitation	FMA (upper limb)	3	264	SMD: 0.89 [0.05, 1.72]*	90	C18, C22, C26
	FMA (lower limb)	3	264	SMD: 0.51 [0.26, 0.75]*	0	C18, C22, C26

*Statistically significant.

Abbreviations: AS – Ashworth Scale; BI – Barthel Index; CHM – Chinese herbal medicine; CI – confidence interval; FMA – Fugl-Meyer Assessment; MAS – Modified Ashworth Scale; MD – mean difference; SMD – standardised mean difference.

Chinese Herbal Medicine plus Acupressure plus Cupping Therapy

One study (C28) including 300 participants, compared the combination of CHM, acupressure, cupping therapy and rehabilitation to rehabilitation alone. It was found that, after one week of treatment, the integrative therapy was more effective than rehabilitation alone for FMA (upper limb) (MD: 3.41 [2.76, 4.06]) and FMA (lower limb) (MD: 4.08 [3.33, 4.83]). However, the study did not report details of the CHM ingredients and acupuncture points. Adverse events data were not reported by this study.

Chinese Herbal Medicine plus *Tuina* 推拿 Therapy

Two studies evaluated the add-on effects of CHM plus *tuina* 推拿 therapy to rehabilitation alone (C8), or to routine care (C20). Both of these studies reported data on FMA (motor function) and MBI. In terms of the FMA (motor function), both studies showed benefit of the integrative therapy, and meta-analysis confirmed the integrative therapy was more effective (MD: 24.95 [23.76, 26.14], $I^2 = 96\%$). With regard to the MBI outcome, although both studies reported a benefit of adding CM therapies, meta-analysis results indicated that there was no difference between the integrative therapy and rehabilitation (MD: 14.61 [–1.85, 31.07], $I^2 = 98\%$). Adverse events data were not reported by these studies.

Comprehensive Chinese Medicine Programme

One study (C16) assessed the add-on therapy of a comprehensive CM programme to routine care. The study applied a comprehensive combination of CM therapies, including oral CHM, CHM bath therapy, acupuncture, ear acupressure, *tuina* 推拿 therapy, moxibustion and CHM diet therapy. All these treatments were selected and tailored according to each patient's syndrome differentiation and symptom severity. In this study, CM therapies were integrated to routine care/rehabilitation, using routine care/rehabilitation as comparator. Our analysis showed that the integrative therapy was more effective than routine care for both MAS (non-specified) (MD: –0.93 [–1.27, –0.59]) and MBI (MD: 8.92 [5.82, 12.02]). In this study, CHM was administered both orally and topically. Acupuncture, moxibustion and *tuina* 推拿 therapy were applied to both the upper and lower limbs. However, the treatment duration was not reported by this study. Adverse events information was not provided.

Evidence for Chinese Medicine Combined Therapies Commonly Used in Clinical Practice

Our search found that many RCTs have evaluated the combinations of different CM therapies including CHM (oral or topical), acupuncture, *tuina* 推拿 therapy and moxibustion for post-stroke spasticity, although none of these combinations were particularly recommended by the clinical guidelines (see Chapter 2 for a summary).

In combination with other CM therapies, two formulas (*Bu yang huan wu tang* 补阳还五汤 and *Zhong feng hui chun wan* 中风回春丸) has been evaluated in multiple RCTs. *Bu yang huan wu tang* 补阳还五汤 is one of the CHM formulas recommended in current clinical guidelines (see Chapter 2). However, meta-analysis for these formulas was not feasible because these studies were not of the same comparison. Single-study results show that, compared to medication (baclofen), oral CHM *Bu yang huan wu tang* 补阳还五汤 plus acupuncture was more effective for patients' motor function (FMA) and daily activity (MBI) (C2). When oral CHM *Bu yang huan wu tang* 补阳还五汤 plus acupuncture was used as an add-on therapy to routine rehabilitation, it also increased treatment effect in terms of patients' motor function (FMA) and daily activity (MBI) (C13).

Acupuncture was recommended by contemporary literature (see Chapter 2), as well as being commonly evaluated by clinical studies. In terms of acupuncture points, there were no 'acupuncture formulas' being assessed in multiple studies. Acupuncture was recommended to focus on needling the antagonistic muscles and to avoid strong stimulation on the muscles with hypertonia or spasticity; such a strategy was also mentioned in most of the clinical studies. *Tuina* 推拿

therapy and moxibustion were also recommended by contemporary literature (see Chapter 2). Our evaluation of clinical studies in this chapter found they were used in combination with CHM or acupuncture.

Summary of Chinese Combined Medicine Therapies Clinical Evidence

This chapter evaluated the combination of two or more CM therapies used as post-stroke spasticity management. Among all included studies, CHM plus acupuncture is the most commonly used combination, followed by the combination of CHM, acupuncture and *tuina* 推拿 therapy. Chinese herbal medicine was the most common therapy and was used by all studies, either orally or topically, or both. Acupuncture (including body acupuncture and scalp acupuncture) was evaluated by 89% of the included studies (25 of 28).

Among the studies investigating the combination of CHM and other therapies, most did not provide standardised formula names. Two formulas (*Bu yang huan wu tang* 补阳还五汤 and *Zhong feng hui chun wan* 中风回春丸) were used in multiple studies; however, their effectiveness could not be confirmed by meta-analysis. The herb ingredients of the formulas are consistent with those frequently used in the studies which only evaluated CHM (see Chapter 5). The most frequently used herbs are *chuan xiong* 川芎, *bai shao/chi shao* 白芍/赤芍, *dan shen* 丹参, *shui zhi* 水蛭, *huang qi* 黄芪, *hong hua* 红花, *gan cao* 甘草, *di long* 地龙, *dang gui* 当归, *tao ren* 桃仁, *hai feng teng* 海风藤 and *mu gua* 木瓜. In particular, *mu gua* 木瓜 is believed to have anti-spasmodic function in the CM concept.

Acupuncture therapy was also commonly used in the included studies. The top ten frequently used acupuncture points are LI4 *Hegu* 合谷, ST5 *Waiguan* 外关, LI11 *Quchi* 曲池, ST36 *Zusanli* 足三里, SP6 *Sanyinjiao* 三阴交, LI10 *Shousanli* 手三里, LI15 *Jianyu* 肩髃, GB34 *Yanglingquan* 阳陵泉, SP9 *Yinlingquan* 阴陵泉, PC6 *Neiguan* 内关 and ST41 *Jiexi* 解溪. These points are often used for treating hemiplegia in clinical practice. In particular, ST41 *Jiexi* 解溪 is often selected to treat spastic equinovarus foot in hemiparetic patients.

Tuina 推拿 therapy was found being used together with other CM therapies. The techniques of *tuina* 推拿 therapy were consistent with those summarised in Chapter 8. Multiple *tuina* 推拿 techniques were applied on muscles or acupuncture points of the limbs with spasticity.

One study (C16) introduced a comprehensive CM programme including oral CHM, CHM bath therapy, acupuncture, ear acupressure, *tuina* 推拿 therapy, moxibustion and CHM diet therapy. All these treatments were selected and tailored according to each patient's syndrome differentiation and severity. This is similar to a 'real-life practice'. Results showed the benefit of adding the CM programme to routine care/rehabilitation for the severity of spasticity (MAS) and patients' daily activities (MBI). However, this study did not introduce details of treatment duration. It is unclear when these treatments were started after a stroke onset and how long they were administered for.

Due to the limited number of included studies, meta-analysis was not feasible for all types of combination therapy. The combinations of CHM plus acupuncture, and CHM plus *tuina* 推拿 therapy had sufficient data to conduct meta-analyses. It was shown that adding CHM and acupuncture to routine care/rehabilitation was beneficial for reducing spasticity of the upper limb (MAS), improving patients' motor function (FMA) and daily activities (MBI). Also, combining CHM and *tuina* 推拿 therapy increased the effectiveness of routine rehabilitation for patients' motor function (FMA). On the other hand, few of the included studies compared combinations of CM interventions with routine care/rehabilitation. There is no meta-analysis evidence showing superior effects of CM combination therapy over routine care/rehabilitation.

Our review of clinical studies did not include the studies comparing two or more CM therapies to one of these therapies (e.g. CHM plus acupuncture versus acupuncture); therefore, it is unclear whether adding more CM therapies is more beneficial then only adding one therapy to routine rehabilitation.

CM combination therapies seem safe for the management of post-stroke spasticity. Based on the evidence of individual CM therapies (see Chapters 5, 7 and 8) and the evidence of combination therapies, practitioners could consider incorporating them into clinical practice.

References to Included Clinical Studies

Study ID	References
C1	孙志英, 韩淑凯, 曹文杰, 刘建会, 左丽卿, 林国群. (2013) 补气化痰通络方结合表里两经并刺法对脑血管病后肩手综合征患者痉挛状态的影响. 陕西中医 **34(8):** 1004–1006.
C2	侯震, 王瑶. (2012) 针药结合对脑卒中后痉挛性偏瘫的疗效观察. 世界中西医结合杂志 **7(4):** 317.
C3	周喜燕, 王雁慧. (2009) 针药结合治疗中风后痉挛性瘫痪的临床观察. 时珍国医国药 **20(4):** 1010–1011.
C4	牛攀东. (2002) 补气活血养肝柔筋针刺补泻治疗脑卒中偏瘫 39 例. 临床中老年保健 **50(1):** 1.
C5	张风林. (2014) 通络牵正方联合针刺治疗中风恢复期神经功能的缺损. 中国实验方剂学杂志 **20(18):** 212–215.
C6	李华, 洪珍梅. (2013) 头针配合超声药物导入治疗中风痉挛性瘫痪 30 例疗效观察. 浙江中医杂志 **48(6):** 448.
C7	许长青, 张凯. (2013) 熏蒸结合针灸治疗中风肢体痉挛 35 例. 中国中医药现代远程教育 **11(2):** 60–61.
C8	王海丽. (2009) 药足浴对脑卒中患者运动功能影响的临床观察. 社区医学杂志 **(11).**
C9	王秀汝. (2012) 早期介入传统中医康复的现代康复治疗对脑卒中后足下垂的疗效观察. 中国现代医学杂志 **(18):** 87–90.
C10	钟如春. (2014) 针刺阿是穴、阴经穴位配合中药治疗脑卒中后肢体痉挛的临床研究. 河南中医 **(11):** 88.
C11	陈华, 周建伟. (2013) 针刺中药康复综合方案预防中风后肢体痉挛的临床研究. 四川中医 **31(11):** 121–125.
C12	朱国祥, 包烨华, 纪晨彤, 邹超. (2004) 针灸结合中药湿热敷治疗中风后上肢高痉挛状态. 针灸临床杂志 **(6):** 17–18.
C13	唐跃富. (2014) 针药结合康复训练的方法对中风偏瘫痉挛状态的康复疗效及安全性评价. 世界中医药 **9(09):** 1218–1220.
C14	聂代数. (2015) 针药联合康复锻炼治疗中风痉挛性偏瘫临床研究. 内蒙古中医药 **34(1):** 26–26.
C15	李连章. (2004) 中风二代回春胶囊结合康复训练治疗脑卒中肢体痉挛的效果评估. 中国临床康复 **(25):** 5320–5321.
C16	刘梨, 余艳兰, 廖若夷, 张月娟. (2013) 中风后痉挛性瘫痪中医护理方案的临床应用. 湖南中医药大学学报 **(9):** 97–101

(*Continued*)

(*Continued*)

Study ID	References
C17	王鹏. (2012) 中风回春丸结合电针治疗中风痉挛性偏瘫. 中国实验方剂学杂志 **(11):** 275–277.
C18	曲红岩, 刘艳芳, 刘智艳. (2014) 中西医结合康复治疗对脑卒中偏瘫痉挛状态的影响. 中医药导报 **07:** 34–36.
C19	银卫华. (2013) 中西医结合治疗中风后偏瘫的临床远期观察. 国际医药卫生导报 **19(05):** 695–697.
C20	冯莉. (2013) 中药熏蒸结合穴位按摩治疗中风痉挛性瘫痪的临床观察. 泸州医学院学报 **34(5):** 523–525.
C21	赵爱英. (2014) 中医康复疗法配合强化步行训练对脑卒中偏瘫患者下肢功能恢复的影响. 河南中医 **34(7):** 1274–1275.
C22	李慧玲. (2015) 中医康复综合疗法应用于偏瘫痉挛状态患者临床干预的应用探析. 中国民康医学 **(6):** 85–87.
C23	陕大艳. (2014) 中医综合康复疗法结合现代康复训练改善中风偏瘫痉挛状态的临床研究. 中医学报 **(08):** 1230–1231.
C24	秦润笋, 赵子龙. (2006) 中医综合康复疗法治疗中风后肌张力增高疗效观察. 辽宁中医杂志 **33(11):** 1456–1457.
C25	陈庆华, 杨丰, 郑红霞. (2008) 综合康复治疗对脑卒中患者运动功能及 ADL 的对照观察. 中国误诊学杂志 **(14):** 3335–3336.
C26	蔡英丽. (2005) 中医综合康复法治疗偏瘫痉挛状态的临床观察. (Thesis). 北京中医药大学.
C27	张娟. (2013) 中西医结合康复方案对脑卒中偏瘫患者生活质量的影响. (Thesis). 广州中医药大学.
C28	韩群英. (2003) 中风病偏瘫中医康复八法的临床研究. (Thesis). 北京中医药大学.

10

Summary and Conclusions

OVERVIEW

Chinese medicine therapies have been used to treat stroke and its complications for a long period in history, including post-stroke hemiplegia and spasticity. This chapter summarises the main findings of the previous chapters, including those from classical literature, modern clinical trial evidence and experimental evidence for the management of post-stroke spasticity. The limitations of the available evidence are discussed, and future directions are identified for further clinical and experimental research.

Introduction

Stroke is currently the leading cause of neurological disability in adults. It can result in high levels of residual disability that can persist for months, years or the remainder of the individual's life. Effective rehabilitation interventions initiated early after stroke can enhance the recovery process and minimise functional disability. Spasticity is one of the most commonly seen motor function problems after stroke. It has been increasingly researched since it may negatively affect rehabilitation outcomes.

Spasticity has been defined as 'disordered sensorimotor control, resulting from an upper motor neuron lesion, presenting as intermittent or sustained involuntary activation of muscles'.[1] It is one of the most significant impairments for stroke survivors, and can result in significant pain and functional disturbances. The most impairing state from spasticity may be contractures, rendering the affected limb with limited function or to become functionless. Skin hygiene may also be a problem with spasticity.[1] In clinical practice, Chinese medicine (CM) therapies usually play the role of assisting conventional therapies in the management of post-stroke spasticity.

In order to provide a 'whole-evidence' evaluation, in this book, we analysed the evidence of CM therapies from all types of literature for post-stroke spasticity. A review of clinical guidelines and textbooks identified a range of CM treatments that have been recommended or suggested for post-stroke spasticity, including oral and topical Chinese herbal medicine (CHM), acupuncture and traditional Chinese *tuina* 推拿 therapy (Chapter 2).

In classical literature, the treatment of post-stroke spasticity was recorded under hemiplegia. Therefore, searches of classical literature were conducted from the angle of overall stroke and post-stroke motor functional impairment (Chapter 3). Numerous clinical trials of CM therapies have been conducted in China. Some of these studies have shown promising results. Using a systematic approach, clinical evidence was found to support the use of CHM (Chapter 5), acupuncture and related therapies (Chapter 7), *tuina* 推拿 therapy (Chapter 8) and some combination of multiple CM therapies (Chapter 9). In general, the herbs and acupuncture points used in these combination therapies were consistent with those used in the studies included in Chapters 5 and 7. Furthermore, the herbs that were used most frequently in the randomised controlled trials (RCTs) have shown actions in experimental studies which shed light on their probable mechanisms of action (Chapter 6).

Chinese Medicine Syndrome Differentiation

According to the CM syndrome differentiation theory, spasticity is considered as a condition with deficiency in the root 本虚 and excess in the superficiality 标实, and closely related to the function of Liver and Kidney organs, *qi* 气 and Blood. The characteristics of the symptoms indicate that spasticity is caused by primarily *yin* 阴 deficiency of the Liver and Kidney resulting in *qi* 气 and Blood deficiency, hence causing the failure of nourishing the tendons (deficiency in the root 本虚), and therefore limb stiffness and contractures occur (excess in the superficiality 标实) (Chapter 2). The treatment principle for post-stroke spasticity is to tonify the Liver and Kidney, nourish *qi* 气 and Blood, soften the tendons and unblock meridians and collaterals.

Syndrome differentiation was not commonly reported in the clinical studies. Only two studies utilising oral CHM considered selecting CHM formulas/herbs according to patients' syndrome differentiation (Chapter 5), which were (1) Wind, Phlegm and Blood stasis blocking the collaterals 风痰瘀血, 痹阻脉络, and (2) *yin* 阴 deficiency with internal Wind 阴虚风动. The syndrome approach was not used in studies evaluating topical CHM (Chapter 5). Similarly, in the 198 studies of acupuncture-related therapies, only eight studies reported information of syndrome, with the most common syndrome seen being 'Liver *yang* uprising, Wind and Phlegm blocking the meridians, with *qi* deficiency and Blood stasis 肝阳上亢, 风痰阻络, 气虚血瘀' (Chapter 7). Also, CM syndrome differentiation seems not essential when applying *tuina* 推拿 therapy for the treatment of post-stroke spasticity since none of the included studies highlighted such information (Chapter 8).

Although the syndrome information was only reported in a small number of studies, the primary syndrome types are consistent with what was suggested in Chapter 2, that is, deficiency in the root and excess in the superficiality 本虚标实. Therefore, clinical treatment should consider using the principle of nourishing *qi* 气 and Blood, tonifying the Liver and Kidney, and unblocking meridians.

Chinese Herbal Medicine

This section summarises the evidence from Chapters 2, 3, 5 and 9. Chinese herbal medicine therapies have been suggested by all forms of evidence in the treatment of post-stroke spasticity. Both oral and topical CHM therapies have been recommended by contemporary textbooks and guidelines, and also evaluated in clinical studies.

Our search of classical literature found more than 200 citations using CHM as treatment for stroke and its motor function impairment, with spasticity-like symptoms specified. The most frequent formulas being introduced in multiple citations were *San huang tang*

三黄汤 (*Qian jin san huang tang* 千金三黄汤), *Xu ming tang* 续命汤, *Xiao xu ming tang* 小续命汤, *Xing feng tang* 省风汤, *Fang feng san* 防风散, *Da jin ya jiu* 大金牙酒, *Zuo jing wan* 左经丸, *Du huo san* 独活散 and *Qin jiao sheng ma tang* 秦艽升麻汤. All these CHM formulas were recorded as being used orally. On the other hand, our search of *Zhong Hua Yi Dian* 中华医典 did not identify any citations with topical CHM. These most frequent CHM formulas found in classical literature are not consistent with those recommended by current clinical guidelines or textbooks (see Chapter 2). Such inconsistency could be explained by the fact that the understanding of stroke's aetiology has changed over time. However, although these formulas are not recommended in contemporary literature for treating post-stroke spasticity, the most frequently used herbs showed the main functions of nourishing Blood and removing Blood stasis, tonifying *qi* 气, Spleen or Kidney, eliminating Wind and unblocking meridians (see Table 3.6 for more information). These functions are similar to the treatment principles used in current practice. Furthermore, it is worth noting that some herbs frequently used historically are no longer in use in current clinical practice. For example, *she xiang* 麝香 is restricted under the provisions of the Convention on International Trade in Endangered Species of Wild Fauna and Flora (CITES). In addition, some herbs, such as *fu zi* 附子, *wu tou* 乌头 and *xi xin* 细辛, may be restricted in some countries due to their toxicity. In fact, the toxicity of *fu zi* 附子 and *wu tou* 乌头 had been noted in classical literature, and certain efforts had been made to reduce their toxicity.

In the evaluation of modern literature data of CHM for post-stroke spasticity, evidence supporting the use of both oral and topical CHM was found (see Chapters 5 and 9). The evidence from meta-analyses for treatment effects showed that oral CHM was an effective add-on therapy for spasticity of the upper and lower limbs (assessed by AS or MAS), overall motor function, upper and lower limbs (assessed by FMA), and patients' daily activities (assessed by BI). Topical CHM had also been shown to be effective when it was used as an add-on therapy for spasticity of the upper and lower limbs (assessed by AS or MAS), overall motor function and upper limbs (assessed by FMA), as well as patients' daily activities (assessed by

BI). In addition, it has been shown by meta-analyses that the combination of oral and topical CHM was also an effective add-on therapy for overall spasticity, motor function and patients' daily activities. Nevertheless, the certainty of most of this evidence was assessed as 'low' or 'very low'. For other outcomes, there were insufficient clinical studies in each category to conduct meta-analyses.

Three orally used CHM formulas (*Bu yang huan wu tang* 补阳还五汤, *Gua lou gui zhi tang* 栝楼桂枝汤 and *Shao yao gan cao tang* 芍药甘草汤), one topically used formula (*Shu jin huo luo xi ji* 舒筋活络洗剂) and another formula being used both orally and topically (*Jie jing he ji* 解痉合剂) had been evaluated in multiple studies. It is worth noting that the oral CHM formula *Bu yang huan wu tang* 补阳还五汤 had not only been repeatedly evaluated in clinical research, but had also been recommended by existing monographs and guidelines. The CHM formula which had been used both orally and topically in clinical research (*Jie jing he ji* 解痉合剂) also contains *shao yao gan cao tang* 芍药甘草汤 as its chief herbs.

Specifically, herbs used orally that may have contributed to the positive effects seen include *bai shao* 白芍, *dang gui* 当归, *gan cao* 甘草, *di long* 地龙 and *huang qi* 黄芪. Among these herbs, *bai shao* 白芍 and *gan cao* 甘草 are the key herbs of the oral CHM formula (*Shao yao gan cao tang* 芍药甘草汤) believed to have the function of relieving muscle spasm. Some herbs are more often used topically, which may have contributed to the positive effects; these are *dang gui* 当归, *mu gua* 木瓜, *shen jin cao* 伸筋草, *bai shao* 白芍 and *chuan xiong* 川芎. Based on these results, practitioners may consider these herbs when preparing prescriptions for patients with post-stroke spasticity, in particular the oral formulas *Bu yang huan wu tang* 补阳还五汤 and *Shao yao gan cao tang* 芍药甘草汤.

Pre-clinical research supports the effects of the most commonly used herbs through neuroprotective, anti-spasmodic and analgesic activities. In particular, the combination of *bai shao* 白芍 and *gan cao* 甘草 (*Shao yao gan cao tang* 芍药甘草汤) has been proven to carry several anti-spasmodic activities. Very few adverse events were reported; however, most of the included studies did not give information of adverse events.

The analysis of treatment effects showed that oral and topical CHM were effective for managing post-stroke spasticity, in particular when they were administered as an effective add-on therapy to conventional rehabilitation and routine care. However, there was considerable variability in the meta-analyses results due to studies of different CHM formulas being pooled together. Currently there has not been sufficient evidence to compare the effects of different formulas. The frequency analysis of CHM formulas and herbs may be able to indicate what are commonly considered in current clinical practice, but without analyses for their efficacy. Other factors influencing the interpretation of the results of the clinical studies were the relatively poor reporting of trial design and methods, and the lack of blinding in most studies. Information of adverse events was not reported in many studies. These aspects reduced confidence in the accuracy of the reported results and resulted in the downgrading of the certainty of the evidence in the Grading of Recommendations Assessment, Development and Evaluation (GRADE) assessments.

Chinese Herbal Medicine Formulas in Key Clinical Guidelines and Textbooks, Classical Literature and Clinical Studies

Table 10.1 summarises the CHM formulas described in clinical guidelines and textbooks (Chapter 2), classical literature (Chapter 3) and clinical studies (Chapter 5). Assessment was based on formula name. It is likely that formulas with the same or similar herb ingredients, but with different formula names, were also included in our evaluation but not shown in this table. As assessment of similarity of formulas is complex and was not undertaken, the actual number for each listed formula may be higher than reported below.

Based on our analysis, the formulas recorded in classical literature are not completely consistent with those being commonly used in current clinical practice. No formula had evidence in all types of literature included in this book. *Bu yang huan wu tang* 补阳还五汤 is the only formula which has been repeatedly evaluated in clinical research, as well as recommended by existing clinical guidelines/textbooks. Furthermore, topical CHM was used in many clinical studies. However, most of these studies did not provide a name for

Table 10.1 Summary of Chinese Herbal Medicine Formulas

Formula Name	Clinical Guidelines and Textbooks (Chapter 2)	Classical Literature (No. of Citations)	Clinical Studies (Chapter 5) (No. of Studies)			Combination Therapies (Chapter 9) (No. of Studies)
			RCTs	CCTs	Non-controlled Studies	
Oral CHM						
Bu yang huan wu tang 补阳还五汤	Yes	0	2	0	0	2
Di huang yin zi 地黄饮子	Yes	0	0	0	0	0
Fu fang tong luo ye 复方通络液	Yes	0	0	0	0	0
Kang jing luan fang 抗痉挛方	Yes	0	0	0	0	0
Gua lou gui zhi tang 栝楼桂枝汤	No	0	2	0	0	0
Shao yao gan cao tang 芍药甘草汤	No	0	2	0	1	0
Topical CHM						
CHM bath therapy: *Fu fang tong luo ye* 复方通络液	Yes	0	0	0	0	0
Kang jing luan fang 抗痉挛方	Yes	0	0	0	0	0
Shu jin huo luo xi ji 舒筋活络洗剂	No	0	2	0	0	0

Abbreviations: CCTs – controlled clinical trials; CHM – Chinese herbal medicine; RCTs – randomised controlled trials.

the formula. It is difficult for clinicians to replicate the clinical research in their practice. Researchers should take this point into consideration in their future work.

Acupuncture and Related Therapies

This section summarises the evidence from Chapters 2, 3, 7 and 9. Overall, consistency was seen in the interventions cited across all evidence types (Table 10.2). Acupuncture therapies have a long

Table 10.2 Summary of Acupuncture and Related Therapies

Acupuncture Therapy	Clinical Guidelines and Textbooks (Chapter 2)	Classical Literature (Chapter 3) (No. of Citations)	Clinical Studies (Chapter 7) (No. of Studies)			Combination Therapies (Chapter 9) (No. of Studies)
			RCTs*	CCTs	Non-controlled Studies	
Body acupuncture	Yes	30	98	11	33	25
Moxibustion	Yes	18	7	0	0	0

*Some studies used more than one intervention e.g. acupuncture plus moxibustion. These are counted separately in this table.

Abbreviations: CCTs – controlled clinical trials; RCTs – randomised controlled trials.

history of use for the clinical management of post-stroke motor function impairment. It is recorded in the classical literature that the use of acupuncture to treat stroke dates back to the Tang dynasty and continues until modern times (Chapter 3). Most of these treatments were found from the books introducing the function of acupuncture points, usually with both acupuncture and moxibustion being applied. In contemporary literature (Chapter 2), in addition to regular acupuncture, a method of applying a moxibustion cone on top of acupuncture needles was recommended as 'warm needling'. Among our evaluation of clinical research, over 160 clinical studies were found having evaluated acupuncture, and seven have evaluated moxibustion.

In addition to the needling acupuncture and moxibustion therapies, some recently developed acupuncture therapies have been investigated in clinical research, including electroacupuncture, scalp acupuncture and acupressure (Chapter 7). It should be noted that an acupuncture technique named *Jin San Zhen* 靳三针 has been evaluated by multiple clinical studies. It seems that this technique has attracted interest for treating post-stroke hemiplegia and spasticity in clinical practice.

In order to summarise which traditional acupuncture points were used for acupuncture and/or moxibustion treatment, all the points that were recommended in Chapter 2 and the points most frequently used in the RCTs in Chapter 7, were included in Table 10.3. The use

Table 10.3 Summary of Acupuncture Points

Acupuncture Point	Clinical Guidelines and Textbooks (Chapter 2)	Classical Literature (Chapter 3) (No. of Citations)	Clinical Studies in Chapter 7 (No. of Studies)			Combination Therapies (Chapter 9) (No. of Studies)
			RCTs	CCTs	Non-controlled Studies*	
Acupuncture						
LI11 *Quchi* 曲池	Yes	7	41	0	11	13
TE5 *Waiguan* 外关	Yes	0	38	5	12	14
LI10 *Shousanli* 手三里	Yes	4	27	4	8	8
GB34 *Yanglingquan* 阳陵泉	Yes	3	25	2	8	8
PC6 *Neiguan* 内关	Yes	2	22	2	8	6
KI6 *Zhaohai* 照海	Yes	0	17	3	2	6
BL40 *Weizhong* 委中	Yes	3	16	2	0	6
TE10 *Tianjing* 天井	Yes	0	12	0	6	0
BL37 *Yinmen* 殷门	Yes	0	12	0	0	1
ST32 *Futu* 伏兔	Yes	0	10	1	1	3
BL57 *Chengshan* 承山	Yes	0	10	1	2	5
TE4 *Yangchi* 阳池	Yes	0	9	0	2	2
ST 34 *Liangqiu* 梁丘	Yes	0	9	0	5	2
ST40 *Fenglong* 丰隆	Yes	0	6	0	4	1
ST37 *Shangjuxu* 上巨虚	Yes	0	5	0	0	0
TE13 *Naohui* 臑会	Yes	0	5	1	3	1
SI9 *Jianzhen* 肩贞	Yes	0	4	0	2	1
TE3 *Zhongzhu* 中渚	Yes	0	4	0	2	1
PC5 *Jianshi* 间使	Yes	0	1	0	0	1
BL39 *Weiyang* 委阳	Yes	0	1	0	0	1
ST33 *Yinshi* 阴市	Yes	0	0	0	0	1
ST36 *Zusanli* 足三里	No	2	25	4	10	13
Moxibustion						
LI11 *Quchi* 曲池	Yes	4	4	0	0	0
LI10 *Shousanli* 手三里	Yes	2	4	0	0	0
GB34 *Yanglingquan* 阳陵泉	Yes	3	2	0	0	0
PC6 *Neiguan* 内关	Yes	0	1	0	0	0

(*Continued*)

Table 10.3 (*Continued*)

Acupuncture Point	Clinical Guidelines and Textbooks (Chapter 2)	Classical Literature (Chapter 3) (No. of Citations)	Clinical Studies in Chapter 7 (No. of Studies)			Combination Therapies (Chapter 9) (No. of Studies)
			RCTs	CCTs	Non-controlled Studies*	
LI4 *Hegu* 合谷	Yes	5	1	0	0	0
SP10 *Xuehai* 血海	Yes	2	1	0	0	0
LU5 *Chize* 尺泽	Yes	0	0	0	0	0
GB30 *Huantiao* 环跳	Yes	4	0	0	0	0
GB31 *Fengshi* 风市	Yes	2	0	0	0	0
GB40 *Qiuxu* 丘墟	Yes	0	0	0	0	0
LR3 *Taichong* 太冲	Yes	0	0	0	0	0

*Some studies used more than one intervention e.g. acupuncture plus moxibustion. These are counted separately in this table.

Abbreviations: CCTs – controlled clinical trials; RCTs – randomised controlled trials.

of these points was cross-referenced to other clinical trial types and other chapters.

All of the points used for acupuncture which were recommended in Chapter 2 have been evaluated in clinical studies, with LI11 *Quchi* 曲池, TE5 *Waiguan* 外关, LI10 *Shousanli* 手三里, GB34 *Yanglingquan* 阳陵泉, PC6 *Neiguan* 内关, KI6 *Zhaohai* 照海, BL40 *Weizhong* 委中, TE10 *Tianjing* 天井, BL37 *Yinmen* 殷门, ST32 *Futu* 伏兔, and BL57 *Chengshan* 承山 being the most common ones. Another acupuncture point, ST36 *Zusanli* 足三里, was also one of the most frequent points in clinical research but it was not included in the contemporary literature we collected and presented (see Chapter 2). In fact, ST36 *Zusanli* 足三里 is also one of the most commonly used points recorded in classical literature.

For the points used for moxibustion, which were recommended in Chapter 2, only six points have been evaluated by clinical studies; they were LI11 *Quchi* 曲池, LI10 *Shousanli* 手三里, GB34 *Yanglingquan* 阳陵泉, PC6 *Neiguan* 内关, LI4 *Hegu* 合谷 and SP10 *Xuehai* 血海. These points have also been recorded in classical literature for moxibustion. The results summarised in Table 10.3 showed consistency of the acupuncture and moxibustion therapies used in classical literature and modern clinical practice.

Other Chinese Medicine Therapies

Tuina 推拿 therapy (Chinese massage) is another type of CM therapy which has been recommended in contemporary texts (Chapter 2) and evaluated in clinical evidence (Chapter 8), but not found in our summary of classical literature (Table 10.4).

In the contemporary literature, *tuina* 推拿 therapy is suggested to be applied on certain acupuncture points located on the upper and lower limbs, using various techniques (Chapter 2). Our evaluation of the clinical evidence indicated that *tuina* 推拿 therapy, when used as an add-on therapy to routine rehabilitation, is beneficial for reducing the severity of upper and lower limb spasticity (assessed by AS or MAS), improving motor function (assessed by FMA), and daily activities (assessed by BI); however, with all evidence being assessed as 'low' certainty. Comparing *tuina* 推拿 therapy itself to routine rehabilitation, results of meta-analysis also indicated superior effects in terms of upper and lower limb spasticity (assessed by AS or MAS).

Clinical research suggested that *tuina* 推拿 therapy was usually applied along meridians, with or without focusing on acupuncture points. Most of the included studies stated that attention should be paid to the strength of applying *tuina* 推拿 therapy on different muscles. A few studies suggested that strong stimulation of the spasm muscles should be avoided. *Tuina* 推拿 therapy could be conducted

Table 10.4 Summary of Other Chinese Medicine Therapy

Other Chinese Medicine Therapy Type	Included in Clinical Guidelines and Textbooks (Chapter 2)	Included in Classical Literature (Chapter 3) (No. of Citations)	Evidence in Clinical Studies (Chapter 8) (No. of Studies)			Included in Combination Therapies (Chapter 9) (No. of Studies)
			RCTs	CCTs	Non-controlled Studies	
Tuina 推拿 therapy	Yes	0	16	1	3	7

Abbreviations: CCTs – controlled clinical trials; RCTs – randomised controlled trials.

daily for 10 to 50 minutes each time. Chinese medicine syndrome differentiation does not seem essential when applying *tuina* 推拿 therapy for the treatment of post-stroke spasticity. It is worth noting that studies with a longer treatment duration (e.g. more than four weeks) reported better treatment effects. Practitioners wishing to use *tuina* 推拿 therapy for post-stroke spasticity should consider this in light of the available evidence.

Limitations of the Evidence

Substantial effort was made in this book to identify data from a wide range of sources; however, there may have been limitations from each of the data resources. Firstly, although spasticity is one of the most commonly seen complications after stroke, it usually is not introduced as an independent condition in contemporary CM clinical guidelines or textbooks. It is common to see literature including anti-spasticity treatment information in the hemiplegia or motor-function impairment sections. Hence, we collected relevant information from various clinical guidelines or textbooks. It is possible that readers may consider that some other treatments are also effective for these complications.

The analyses of the classical literature (Chapter 3) were based on the large sample of CM books which are included in *Zhong Hua Yi Dian* 中华医典 Version 5. Our assessments indicated that this was the largest available digital resource at the time but it did not include every CM book published in pre-modern eras so omissions were unavoidable. We identified a number of different search terms for the search process of *Zhong Hua Yi Dian* 中华医典, but it is not certain that all relevant citations were located and included in the analyses. On the other hand, considering the citations were written by multiple individuals over history, the language usage and meaning of those terms have changed over time. Therefore, the citations located by these terms may carry slightly inconsistent implications. Similarly, the identity of some herbs can change over time and with geographical position, so it is possible that regularisation errors have been made in the allocation of scientific names. Moreover, considering there has not been any disease name referring to post-stroke spasticity, the analyses of CM treatment in classical literature were based on symptoms of post-stroke motor function impairment in combination with the presence of spasticity-like symptoms. While the understanding of stroke aetiology and pathogenesis in history has developed from external pathogen to 'internal Wind', the CM treatment principle also switched from eliminating external Wind to removing Blood stasis. Therefore, the results of our analyses calculating the frequently used herbs may not be completely consistent with those in current use. Also, it is not accurate to assume that the most frequently used herbs represent the most effective treatments because there is no method to evaluate the efficacy. What they represent is a short list of herbs that could be considered for further research.

The clinical trial evidence was based on the search of multiple databases and resulted in thousands of search results. Since there was considerable variation in the conditions under which these trials were conducted, the age and severity of the participants, the frequency and duration of interventions, and the procedures used in data collection and analysis, it was not surprising that statistical heterogeneity tended to be high, although random effects models were used. Where possible, subgroup analyses were conducted but they did not reduce the heterogeneity. The quality of the reporting of the methodological details of trial design and conduct was not adequate in many studies. Most of included studies did not report proper random sequence generation. Blinding had not been applied and there was inadequate information on drop-outs in the majority of studies. In some chapters, clinical evidence sometimes showed inconsistent results across different outcome measures, in particular the outcomes of the upper or lower limb. It is difficult to discover the causes of such diversity. The small number of studies included in each meta-analysis could be one of the reasons; future research is needed to confirm our results.

For each category of evidence, frequency tables are provided that summarise the most commonly used interventions including the herbal formula names, the herbal ingredients used in the formulas and the acupuncture points used in the clinical studies. Due to the large volume of available data, presentation of the details of every study was not feasible and these tables only include the interventions that were the most frequently used. Lower frequency interventions may not be mentioned unless these featured prominently in the meta-analyses. Also, it should not be inferred that the most frequently used interventions were the most effective ones.

Although there are over 300 clinical studies included in our evaluation, only two RCTs investigating the treatment effects of acupuncture were conducted outside China. All other clinical studies were conducted in hospitals in China and recruited patients of Chinese populations only. It is not surprising that those patients who were admitted in hospitals in China may hold high expectations toward CM therapies. The majority of included clinical studies compared the combination of CM therapy with routine care/rehabilitation, to routine care/rehabilitation alone. In such studies, there was often a benefit for the combination therapy, particularly when no placebo for the CM therapy was used, and the patients were not blinded for their group allocation. Therefore, when CM therapies were used as an add-on therapy to routine care/rehabilitation, the treatment effects may have been inflated due to the belief of their effects in Chinese culture. In addition, only a small number of studies included a follow-up phase to evaluate the long-term effects of CM therapies. Considering that spasticity causes long-term impacts on patients' activities and affects patients' quality of life, evaluating long-term treatment effects is important for providing evidence to clinical practice.

It is noted that adverse events have not been reported in detail by most of the included studies, showing that the clinical research conducted in China has not paid enough attention to evaluating the safety of CM therapies. Future research should also improve the quality in this aspect. The above limitations should be taken into consideration when interpreting the data included in the previous chapters.

Implications for Practice

Traditionally, CM practice has been inherited from the records in previous literature or senior practitioners' clinical experience.

The evidence-based practice approach was not adopted for the development of textbooks or clinical practice guidelines in CM. In this book, we evaluated evidence from classical literature and current clinical research, and provided information on how, and to what extent, treatments of post-stroke spasticity were developed. The research provides evidence which supports the recommendation for use of CM therapies and identified the gap between contemporary literature and current clinical practice in terms of some treatment methods.

In history, post-stroke spasticity was not addressed as an independent clinical condition. Therefore, relevant treatments were identified from the citations of stroke (*zhong feng* 中风) which had spasticity-like symptoms being mentioned. The word *zhong feng* 中风 refers to 'a sudden Wind attack'. The concept of 'Wind' in stroke was initially an external pathogen which then developed to being internal factors. As a result, CHM formulas and herbs, which have the function of eliminating external Wind, appeared as the commonly used ones in our frequency analyses.

The clinical trial evidence, in particular the evidence from RCTs, provides the best available evidence for the effectiveness of particular CM interventions. Our evaluation of current clinical studies indicated that adding CM therapies to routine care/rehabilitation is generally beneficial for relieving the severity of spasticity, and improving patients' motor function and daily activities. Findings from reviews of clinical evidence suggest that CHM, acupuncture therapies and *tuina* 推拿 therapy could be incorporated into an overall health care plan for post-stroke spasticity, in particular being used as add-on therapies to routine care and rehabilitation. The certainty of evidence had been assessed for the main therapies using the GRADE approach. It was found that:

- Oral CHM, topical CHM, and oral plus topical CHM were effective add-on therapies (GRADE: 'Very low' to 'low');
- Acupuncture, electroacupuncture and acupressure were effective add-on therapies (GRADE: 'Very low' to 'low');
- *Tuina* 推拿 therapy was an effective add-on therapy (GRADE: 'Low').

There is more clinical evidence supporting the use of oral CHM than topical CHM. When oral CHM is used in combination with routine care/rehabilitation, it could reduce patients' spasticity, and improve motor function and daily activities. The average treatment duration is one month. Two CHM formulas could be highlighted from our analyses of current clinical studies (*Bu yang huan wu tang* 补阳还五汤 and *Shao yao gan cao tang* 芍药甘草汤). Topical CHM can be applied as steaming therapy, heat pack or paste for topical application. Topical CHM is also applied in combination with routine care/rehabilitation, for an average of a one-month treatment duration. Herbs used orally which may have contributed to the positive meta-analyses results were *bai shao* 白芍, *dang gui* 当归, *di long* 地龙, *huang qi* 黄芪 and *shen jin cao* 伸筋草, while those used topically were *hong hua* 红花, *dang gui* 当归 and *chuan xiong* 川芎.

Acupuncture and moxibustion therapies have been consistently recorded in all forms of literature. Clinical evidence also showed the benefit of some modern-style acupuncture therapies, although they were not mentioned in classical literature or clinical guidelines. Acupuncture or electroacupuncture, when used in combination with routine care/rehabilitation, can reduce the severity of spasticity, and improve patients' motor function and daily activities. The treatment duration is, on average, 34 days. Acupressure and moxibustion are also effective for reducing spasticity severity and improving patients' motor function and daily activities, with the average duration being seven weeks and one month, respectively. The acupuncture points used for body acupuncture, which possibly have contributed to the positive meta-analyses results, were LI4 *Hegu* 合谷, SP6 *Sanyinjiao* 三阴交, SJ5 *Waiguan* 外关, LI11 *Quchi* 曲池, ST36 *Zusanli* 足三里, LU5 *Chize* 尺泽 and SP9 *Yinlingquan* 阴陵泉, while those used for electroacupuncture were LI4 *Hegu* 合谷, SJ5 *Waiguan* 外关, LI10 *Shousanli* 手三里, LI11 *Quchi* 曲池, GB34 *Yanglingquan* 阳陵泉, SP6 *Sanyinjiao* 三阴交 and ST36 *Zusanli* 足三里. Clinicians should use their clinical judgment when considering these techniques for people with post-stroke spasticity.

Tuina 推拿 therapy seems to play an important role in the management of post-stroke spasticity. It was proved that combining *tuina* 推拿 therapy with routine care/rehabilitation was beneficial for reducing spasticity severity and improving patients' motor function and daily activities, with an average duration of 38 days. *Tuina* 推拿 therapy can be applied for 30 minutes each time, focusing on paralysed muscles or local meridians/points. When applying *tuina* 推拿 therapy in clinical practice, a special precaution should be taken, that is, strong stimulation of the spasm muscles should be avoided.

Implications for Research

Chinese medicine therapies are increasingly evaluated through clinical trials, in line with the development of western medicine. Our systematic analyses of modern literature and classical literature have provided a list of herbs and acupuncture points that have been used in the clinical literature related to the management of post-stroke spasticity. Future experimental studies will improve the understanding of their mechanisms of action and may lead to new therapeutic agents.

Although our systematic analyses found that CM management of post-stroke spasticity is consistent and encouraging, high-certainty evidence is lacking. Hence, there is a need for well-designed clinical trials of CM interventions in order to provide accurate assessment of treatment effects. Rigorous methodology is needed when designing future clinical trials of CM therapies in this area; in particular, attention should be paid to adequate randomisation and allocation concealment.

Considering that the CM therapies commonly are administered as add-on therapies to routine care/rehabilitation, efforts should be made to ensure blinding of participants and practitioner with the use of placebo or sham control. Although for acupuncture and other manual therapies, the difficulties in blinding the person delivering the therapy are well-known, it is feasible to blind the participants using a sham device.[2–4]

With regard to the outcome measures, the use of MAS for assessing spasticity severity should be standardised. Currently there are different scaling methods being used in clinical research, making our meta-analyses for overall effects challenging. Since these results were presented with standard mean difference, the minimum detectable difference of MAS could not be used to explain the results. Since post-stroke spasticity is a long-term condition, long-term effects of CM therapies should be evaluated in the follow-up phase using well-validated outcome measures.

Diversity was seen in the range of CM therapies, both within and across forms of evidence, reflecting the nature of CM clinical practice. Future research should focus on the most promising findings identified and investigate the efficacy and safety of those therapies that are feasible to be widely used in clinical practice.

References

1. Duncan PW, Zorowitz R, Bates B, *et al.* (2005) Management of adult stroke rehabilitation care: A clinical practice guideline. *Stroke* **36(9):** e100–e143.
2. Zhang CS, Yang AW, Zhang AL, *et al.* (2014) Sham control methods used in ear-acupuncture/ear-acupressure randomized controlled trials: A systematic review. *J Altern Complement Med* **20(3):** 147–161.
3. Zhang CS, Tan HY, Zhang GS, *et al.* (2015) Placebo devices as effective control methods in acupuncture clinical trials: A systematic review. *PLoS One* **10(11):** e0140825.
4. Zhang GS, Zhang CS, Tan HY, *et al.* (2018) Systematic review of acupuncture placebo devices with a focus on the credibility of blinding of healthy participants and/or acupuncturists. *Acupunct Med* **36(4):** 204–214.

Glossary

Terms	Acronym	Definition	Reference
95% confidence interval	95% CI	A measure of the uncertainty around the main finding of a statistical analysis. Estimates of unknown quantities, such as the odds ratio comparing an experimental intervention with a control, are usually presented as a point estimate and a 95% confidence interval. This means that if someone were to keep repeating a study in other samples from the same population, 95% of the confidence intervals from those studies would contain the true value of the unknown quantity. Alternatives to 95%, such as 90% and 99% confidence intervals, are sometimes used. Wider intervals indicate lower precision; narrow intervals, greater precision.	http://handbook.cochrane.org/
Acupressure	—	Application of pressure to acupuncture points.	—
Acupuncture	—	The insertion of needles into humans or animals for remedial purposes.	World Health Organisation. (2007) WHO International Standard Terminologies of Traditional Medicine in the Western Pacific Region.
Allied and Complementary Medicine Database	AMED	Alternative medicine bibliographic database.	https://www.ebscohost.com/academic/AMED-The-Allied-and-Complementary-Medicine-Database

(*Continued*)

(*Continued*)

Terms	Acronym	Definition	Reference
Ashworth Scale	AS	An outcome measure to assess the severity of spasticity (the amount of resistance or tone perceived by the examiner as a limb is moved through its full range of motion).	—
Barthel Index	BI	A simple tool for assessing self-care and mobility, consisting of ten common activities of daily living, administered through direct observation.	—
China National Knowledge Infrastructure	CNKI	Chinese language bibliographic database.	www.cnki.net
Chinese Biomedical Literature database	CBM	Chinese language bibliographic database.	https://cbmwww.imicams.ac.cn
Chinese herbal medicine	CHM	Chinese herbal formulation	—
Chongqing VIP Information Company	CQVIP	Chinese language bibliographic database.	www.cqvip
ClinicalTrials.gov	—	Clinical trial registry.	https://clinicaltrials.gov/
Cochrane Central Register of Controlled Trials	CENTRAL	Bibliographic database that provides a highly concentrated source of reports of randomised controlled trials.	https://community.cochrane.org/editorial-and-publishing-policy-resource/overview-cochrane-library-and-related-content/databases-included-cochrane-library/cochrane-central-register-controlled-trials-central
Combination therapies	—	Two or more Chinese medicines from different therapy groups (CHM, acupuncture therapies or other CM therapies) administered together.	—

(*Continued*)

(*Continued*)

Terms	Acronym	Definition	Reference
Convention on International Trade in Endangered Species of Wild Fauna and Flora	CITES	International convention aimed at preventing or regulating trade in threatened and endangered species of plants and animals.	https://www.cites.org/eng/disc/text.php
Cumulative Index of Nursing and Allied Health Literature	CINAHL	Bibliographic database.	https://www.ebscohost.com/nursing/about
Cupping therapy	—	Suction by using a vacuumised cup or jar.	World Health Organisation. (2007) WHO International Standard Terminologies of Traditional Medicine in the Western Pacific Region.
Effect size	—	A generic term for the estimate of effect of treatment for a study.	http://handbook.cochrane.org/
Effective rate	ER	A measure of the proportion of participants who achieved an improvement, as outlined in the methods for evaluating clinical evidence section.	—
Electroacupuncture	—	Electric stimulation of the needle following insertion.	World Health Organisation. (2007) WHO International Standard Terminologies of Traditional Medicine in the Western Pacific Region.
Excerpta Medica database	Embase	Bibliographic database.	http://www.elsevier.com/solutions/embase
Fugl-Meyer Assessment	FMA	A disease-specific impairment index designed to assess motor function, balance, sensation qualities and joint function in hemiplegic post-stroke patients.	—
Grading of Recommendations Assessment, Development and Evaluation	GRADE	Approach to grading quality of evidence and strength of recommendations.	http://www.gradeworkinggroup.org/

(*Continued*)

(*Continued*)

Terms	Acronym	Definition	Reference
Heterogeneity	—	1. Used in a general sense to describe the variation in, or diversity of, participants, interventions, and measurement of outcomes across a set of studies, or the variation in internal validity of those studies. 2. Used specifically, as statistical heterogeneity, to describe the degree of variation in the effect estimates from a set of studies. Also used to indicate the presence of variability among studies beyond the amount expected due solely to the play of chance.	http://handbook.cochrane.org/
I^2	—	A measure of study heterogeneity; indicates the percentage of variance in a meta-analysis.	http://handbook.cochrane.org/
Mean difference	MD	In meta-analysis, a method used to combine measures on continuous scales, where the mean, standard deviation and sample size in each group are known. The weight given to the difference in means from each study (e.g. how much influence each study has on the overall results of the meta-analysis) is determined by the precision of its estimate of effect; mathematically this is equal to the inverse of the variance. This method assumes that all of the trials have measured the outcome on the same scale.	http://handbook.cochrane.org/
Meta-analysis	—	The use of statistical techniques in a systematic review to integrate the results of included studies. Sometimes misused as a synonym for systematic reviews, where the review includes a meta-analysis.	—

(*Continued*)

(*Continued*)

Terms	Acronym	Definition	Reference
Modified Ashworth Scale	MAS	An outcome measure to assess the severity of spasticity (the amount of resistance or tone perceived by the examiner as a limb is moved through its full range of motion).	—
Modified Barthel Index	MBI	Measure of physical disability used widely to assess behaviour relating to activities of daily living for stroke patients or patients with other disabling conditions. It measures what patients do in practice. Assessment is made by anyone who knows the patient well.	—
Moxibustion	—	A therapeutic procedure involving ignited material (usually moxa) to apply heat to certain points or areas of the body surface for curing disease through regulation of the function of meridians/channels and visceral organs.	World Health Organisation. (2007) WHO International Standard Terminologies of Traditional Medicine in the Western Pacific Region.
Non-controlled studies	—	Observations made on individuals, usually receiving the same intervention, before and after an intervention but with no control group.	http://handbook.cochrane.org/
Non-randomised controlled clinical trials	CCT	An experimental study in which people are allocated to different interventions using methods that are not random.	http://handbook.cochrane.org/
Other Chinese medicine therapies	—	Other Chinese medicine therapies include all traditional therapies except Chinese herbal medicine and acupuncture, such as *tai chi* 太极, *qigong* 气功, Chinese pulmonary rehabilitation, *tuina* 推拿 and cupping.	—
PubMed	PubMed	Bibliographic database.	http://www.ncbi.nlm.nih.gov/pubmed
Randomised controlled trial	RCT	Clinical trial that uses a random method to allocate participants to treatment and control groups.	—
Range of motion	ROM	—	—

(*Continued*)

(*Continued*)

Terms	Acronym	Definition	Reference
Risk of bias	—	Assessment of clinical trials to indicate if the results may overestimate or underestimate the true effect because of bias in study design or reporting.	http://handbook.cochrane.org/
Risk ratio	RR	The ratio of risks in two groups. In intervention studies, it is the ratio of the risk in the intervention group to the risk in the control group. A risk ratio of 1 indicates no difference between comparison groups. For undesirable outcomes, a risk ratio that is less than 1 indicates that the intervention was effective in reducing the risk of that outcome.	http://handbook.cochrane.org/
Standardised mean difference	SMD	In meta-analysis, a method used to combine results for continuous scales which measure the same outcome, but it in different ways (e.g. with different scales). The results of studies are standardised to a uniform scale to allow data to be combined.	http://handbook.cochrane.org/
Summary of findings	SoF	Presentation of results and rating the quality of evidence based on the GRADE approach.	http://www.gradeworkinggroup.org/
Tuina 推拿	—	Chinese massage: rubbing, kneading or percussion of the soft tissues and joints of the body with the hands, usually performed by one person on another, especially to relieve tension or pain.	World Health Organisation. (2007) WHO International Standard Terminologies of Traditional Medicine in the Western Pacific Region.
Visual analogue scale	VAS	A commonly used unidimensional measurement instrument to measure pain intensity.	—
Wanfang database	Wanfang	Chinese language bibliographic database.	www.wanfangdata.com

(*Continued*)

(*Continued*)

Terms	Acronym	Definition	Reference
World Health Organisation	WHO	WHO is the directing and coordinating authority for health within the United Nations system. It is responsible for providing leadership on global health matters, shaping the health research agenda, setting norms and standards, articulating evidence-based policy options, providing technical support to countries and monitoring and assessing health trends.	http://www.who.int/about/en/
Zhong Hua Yi Dian 中华医典	ZHYD	The *Zhong Hua Yi Dian* (ZHYD) [*Encyclopaedia of Traditional Chinese Medicine*] is a comprehensive series of electronic books on compact disk. The collection was put together by the Hunan electronic and audio-visual publishing house. It is the largest collection of Chinese electronic books and includes the major Chinese classical works, many of which are from rare manuscripts and are the only existing copies. These books cover the period from before the Tang dynasty to the period of the Republic of China (1911–1948).	Hu R, ed. (2014) *Zhong Hua Yi Dian* [*Encyclopaedia of Traditional Chinese Medicine*], 5th ed. Hunan Electronic and Audio-Visual Publishing House, Chengsha.
Zhong Yi Fang Ji Da Ci Dian 中医方剂大辞典	ZYFJDCD	Compendium of Chinese herbal formulas with over 96,592 entries derived from classical Chinese books. The Nanjing Chinese Medicine Institute compiled the ZYFJDCD and first published it in 1993.	Peng HR, ed. (1994) *Zhong Yi Fang Ji Da Ci Dian* [*Great Compendium of Chinese Medical Formulae*]. People's Medical Publishing House, Beijing.

Index

Evidence-based Clinical Chinese Medicine

Print ISSN: 2529-7562
Online ISSN: 2529-7554

Published

Vol. 1 *Chronic Obstructive Pulmonary Disease*
by Charlie Changli Xue and Chuanjian Lu

Vol. 2 *Psoriasis Vulgaris*
Lead Authors: Claire Shuiqing Zhang and Jingjie Yu

Vol. 3 *Chronic Urticaria*
Lead Authors: Meaghan Coyle and Jingjie Yu

Vol. 4 *Adult Asthma*
Lead Authors: Johannah Shergis and Lei Wu

Vol. 5 *Allergic Rhinitis*
Lead Authors: Claire Shuiqing Zhang and Qiulan Luo

Vol. 6 *Herpes Zoster and Post-herpetic Neuralgia*
Lead Authors: Meaghan Coyle and Haiying Liang

Vol. 7 *Insomnia*
Lead Authors: Johannah Shergis and Xiaojia Ni

Vol. 8 *Alzheimer's Disease*
Lead Authors: Brian H May and Mei Feng

Vol. 9 *Vascular Dementia*
Lead Authors: Brian H May and Mei Feng

Vol. 10 *Diabetic Kidney Disease*
Lead Authors: Johannah Shergis and Lihong Yang

Vol. 11 *Acne Vulgaris*
Lead Authors: Meaghan Coyle and Haiying Liang

More information on this series can also be found at https://www.worldscientific.com/series/ebccm

Vol. 12 *Post-Stroke Shoulder Complications*
Lead Authors: Claire Shuiqing Zhang and Shaonan Liu

Vol. 13 *Post-Stroke Spasticity*
Lead Authors: Claire Shuiqing Zhang and Shaonan Liu

Vol. 14 *Unipolar Depression*
Lead Authors: Yuan Ming Di and Lingling Yang

Vol. 15 *Chronic Heart Failure*
Lead Authors: Claire Shuiqing Zhang and Liuling Ma

Vol. 16 *Atopic Dermatitis*
Lead Authors: Meaghan Coyle and Junfeng Liu

Vol. 17 *Colorectal Cancer*
Lead Authors: Brian H May and Yihong Liu

Forthcoming

Vol. 20 *Chronic Cough*
Lead Authors: Johannah Shergis and Yuanbin Chen

Vol. 22 *Urinary Tract Infection*
Lead Authors: Meaghan Coyle and Xindong Qin

Vol. 24 *Menopause*
Lead Authors: Meaghan Coyle and Jian Liu

Lightning Source UK Ltd.
Milton Keynes UK
UKHW020733190720
366756UK00001B/22

9 789811 213717